Building Innovative Nurse Leaders at the Point of Care

Editor

KELLY A. WOLGAST

NURSING CLINICS OF NORTH AMERICA

www.nursing.theclinics.com

Consulting Editor
STEPHEN D. KRAU

March 2020 • Volume 55 • Number 1

ELSEVIER

1600 John F. Kennedy Boulevard • Suite 1800 • Philadelphia, Pennsylvania, 19103-2899

http://www.theclinics.com

NURSING CLINICS OF NORTH AMERICA Volume 55, Number 1
March 2020 ISSN 0029-6465, ISBN-13: 978-0-323-69567-1

Editor: Kerry Holland
Developmental Editor: Casey Potter

Nursing Clinics of North America (ISSN 0029-6465) is published quarterly by Elsevier Inc., 360 Park Avenue South, New York, NY 10010-1710. Months of issue are March, June, September, and December. Periodicals postage paid at New York, NY and additional mailing offices. Subscription price per year is, $163.00 (US individuals), $518.00 (US institutions), $275.00 (international individuals), $631.00 (international institutions), $231.00 (Canadian individuals), $631.00 (Canadian institutions), $100.00 (US and Canadian students), and $135.00 (international students). To receive student/resident rate, orders must be accompanied by name of affiliated institution, date of term, and the signature of program/residency coordinator on institution letterhead. Orders will be billed at individual rate until proof of status is received. Foreign air speed delivery is included in all *Clinics* subscription prices. All prices are subject to change without notice. **POSTMASTER:** Send address changes to *Nursing Clinics*, Elsevier Health Sciences Division, Subscription Customer Service, 3251 Riverport Lane, Maryland Heights, MO 63043. **Customer Service: Telephone: 1-800-654-2452** (U.S. and Canada); **1-314-447-8871 (outside U.S. and Canada). Fax: 1-314-447-8029. E-mail: journalscustomerservice-usa@ elsevier.com** (for print support) and **journalsonlinesupport-usa@elsevier.com** (for online support).

Nursing Clinics of North America is covered in *EMBASE/Excerpta Medica, MEDLINE/PubMed (Index Medicus), Social Sciences Citation Index, Current Contents, ASCA, Cumulative Index to Nursing, RNdex Top 100,* and Allied Health Literature and International Nursing Index (INI).

Contributors

CONSULTING EDITOR

STEPHEN D. KRAU, PhD, RN, CNE
Associate Professor (Ret), Vanderbilt University School of Nursing, Nashville, Tennessee

EDITOR

KELLY A. WOLGAST, DNP, RN, FACHE, FAAN
Colonel (R), US Army, Associate Teaching Professor, Assistant Dean for Online Education and Outreach, College of Nursing, The Pennsylvania State University, University Park, Pennsylvania

AUTHORS

MARIANNE ADAM, PhD, RN, CRNP
Associate Teaching Professor, College of Nursing, The Pennsylvania State University, Schuylkill Haven, Pennsylvania

LUCY ADAMS
Sophomore Honor's Nursing Student, College of Nursing, The Pennsylvania State University, Scranton Campus, Dunmore, Pennsylvania

KATHERINE ANDREWS, MSN, RN, CCRN
Clinical Nurse, Surgical Intensive Care Unit, Thomas Jefferson University Hospital, Philadelphia, Pennsylvania

ALICIA A. BERGMAN, PhD
Research Health Scientist, VA Health Services Research and Development Center for the Study of Healthcare Innovation, Implementation and Policy, VA Greater Los Angeles Healthcare System, North Hills, California

LORRAINE BOCK, DNP, FNP-C, ENP-C, FAANP
Assistant Teaching Professor, College of Nursing, The Pennsylvania State University, Hershey, Pennsylvania

SARAH E. BRADLEY, MA
Health Science Specialist, Rehabilitation Outcomes Research Section, James A. Haley Veterans' Hospital and Clinics, Tampa, Florida

PETER BUCKLAND, PhD
Penn State's Sustainability Institute, Academic Programs Manager, Affiliate Faculty, Educational Theory and Policy, University Park, Pennsylvania

ASHLEY CLARK, DNP, RN
Assistant Teaching Professor, College of Nursing, The Pennsylvania State University, University Park, Pennsylvania

DARLENE CLARK, MS, RN
Assistant Teaching Professor, College of Nursing, The Pennsylvania State University, University Park, Pennsylvania

MICHAEL M. EVANS, PhD, MSEd, RN, ACNS, CMSRN, CNE
Assistant Dean for Undergraduate Nursing Education at the Commonwealth Campuses, Associate Teaching Professor of Nursing, College of Nursing, The Pennsylvania State University, Scranton Campus, Dunmore, Pennsylvania

JACQUELINE FICKEL, PhD
Research Health Scientist, VA Health Services Research and Development Center for the Study of Healthcare Innovation, Implementation and Policy, VA Greater Los Angeles Healthcare System, North Hills, California

MARGUERITE FLEMING, MPA
Management Analyst, Veterans Health Administration, VA Office of Reporting, Analytics, Performance, Improvement, and Deployment, Washington, DC

KRISTAL HOCKENBERRY, MSN, RN
Simulation Laboratory Coordinator, Nursing Instructor, College of Nursing, The Pennsylvania State University, University Park, Pennsylvania

DIANE JANKURA, MA
Graduate Programs Adviser, Recruitment Coordinator, College of Nursing, The Pennsylvania State University, State College, Pennsylvania

MARY LOUISE KANASKIE, PhD, RN-BC
Director, Office of Nursing Research and Innovation, Penn State Health Milton S. Hershey Medical Center, Hershey, Pennsylvania; Assistant Professor of Nursing and Public Health Sciences, The Pennsylvania State University, University Park, Pennsylvania

JUDITH R. KATZBURG, PhD, MPH, RN
Health Science Specialist, VA Health Services Research and Development, VA Greater Los Angeles Healthcare System, North Hills, California

ERIN KITT-LEWIS, PhD, RN
Assistant Research Professor, College of Nursing, The Pennsylvania State University, University Park, Pennsylvania

JANET KNOTT, DNP, RN, CNE
College of Nursing, The Pennsylvania State University, Assistant Teaching Professor, Penn State New Kensington, New Kensington, Pennsylvania

KALÉI KOWALCHIK
Senior Honor's Nursing Student, Undergraduate, Graduate Research Assistant, College of Nursing, The Pennsylvania State University, Scranton Campus, Dunmore, Pennsylvania

LEON B. LEE, MA
Program Support Assistant, VA Health Services Research and Development Center for the Study of Healthcare Innovation, Implementation and Policy, VA Greater Los Angeles Healthcare System, Los Angeles, California

JASON D. LIND, PhD, MPH
Research Health Science Specialist, Rehabilitation Outcomes Research Section, James A. Haley Veterans' Hospital and Clinics, Tampa, Florida

MARIE ANN MARINO, EdD, RN, FAAN
Dean and Professor, Thomas Jefferson University College of Nursing, Philadelphia, Pennsylvania

SHERI MATTER, PhD, RN, MSN, MBA, MS, NEA-BC
Assistant Teaching Professor, College of Nursing, The Pennsylvania State University, University Park, Pennsylvania

NICOLE MAZUR, MSN, RN
Mount Nittany Medical Center, State College, Pennsylvania

DELORES (DEDE) J. McCREARY, DNP, RN, CNE
Associate Teaching Professor, Nursing, The Pennsylvania State University, Altoona, Pennsylvania

SARAH E. McVEIGH, DNP, GCNS-BC, RN
Nursing Instructor, College of Nursing, University of Iowa, Iowa City, Iowa

ASHLEY MEKIS, MSN, RN, OCN, NE-BC
Mount Nittany Medical Center, State College, Pennsylvania

CAROLE R. MYERS, PhD, RN, FAAN
Professor, University of Tennessee, College of Nursing, Knoxville, Tennessee

MARY ALYCE NELSON, DNP, RN
Assistant Teaching Professor, College of Nursing, The Pennsylvania State University, University Park, Pennsylvania

MICHAEL K. ONG, MD, PhD
VA Health Services Research and Development Center for the Study of Healthcare Innovation, Implementation and Policy, VA Greater Los Angeles Healthcare System, Associate Professor, Department of Medicine, David Geffen School of Medicine at UCLA, Department of Health Policy and Management, UCLA Fielding School of Public Health, Los Angeles, California

KRISTINE A. REYNOLDS, MSN, RN
Magnet Program Director, Penn State Health Milton S. Hershey Medical Center, Hershey, Pennsylvania

KIERNAN RILEY, BSN, RN
BSN to PhD Student, University Fellow, College of Nursing, The Pennsylvania State University, University Park Campus, State College, Pennsylvania

DIANE COWPER RIPLEY, PhD
Advisory Board Member, Veterans Rural Health Resource Center, VA Medical Center, Gainesville, Florida

SARAH A. TUBBESING, MD, MSc
Medical Director, VA Greater Los Angeles Healthcare System Home-Based Primary Care Program, VA Greater Los Angeles Healthcare System, Assistant Professor, Department of Medicine, David Geffen School of Medicine at UCLA, Los Angeles, California

JULIA WARD, PhD, RN
Department Chair - Undergraduate Nursing, Assistant Professor, Thomas Jefferson University College of Nursing, Philadelphia, Pennsylvania

KELLY A. WOLGAST, DNP, RN, FACHE, FAAN
Colonel (R), US Army, Associate Teaching Professor, Assistant Dean for Online Education and Outreach, College of Nursing, The Pennsylvania State University, University Park, Pennsylvania

Contents

> Emerging nurse leaders are not adequately prepared to handle the pervasive health care problems and threats related to the changing environment. Nurse educators prepare nurses for an extensive variety of roles and responsibilities necessary to meet the health care needs of society. The Penn State College of Nursing implemented several initiatives to support environmental sustainability within the college and nursing education. The inclusion of environmental sustainability in nursing education is foundational if students are to become informed members and emerging leaders of a broader health care team, advocates for conscientious and ethical resource use, and contributors to improved patient outcomes.

> Nurses need to actively embrace strategies to improve population health outcomes and reduce health and other disparities. Effective strategies include a focus on the broad range of factors and conditions that have a strong influence on health, advocacy directed at reducing barriers to improved population health, and engagement in policy making. Media engagement is an important tool for amplifying messages about societal problems amenable to public policy, educating stakeholders, bringing diverse stakeholders together for a common purpose, and promoting policy change.

> Nurse bedside shift report (NBSR) focuses on patient-centered care, and implementing the change starts with buy-in from management and a strong educational platform. Based on that platform, nurse champions grow to help foster education to their peers. Education and tools were provided to Registered Nurses and Certified Nursing Assistants. The pilot was implemented in 2 phases onto the Medical Oncology unit, and an incentive program ran concurrently. A prepilot revealed the following projected barriers: time to complete NBSR, concerns with the Health Insurance

Portability and Accountability Act, attending to patient needs, and being able to perform NBSR.

The complexity and rapidly changing environment of health care places significant pressure on nurses. How nurses make decisions within this environment has been an area of inquiry in the literature. Clinical decision making is the application of distinct thinking patterns and analysis of data at hand used to make judgements about patient care. Models of clinical decision making provide a foundation for understanding how nurses make decisions. Key factors associated with clinical decision making include experience, intuition, use of information and sources, and environment. Further work is needed to increase understanding of the processes by which nurses make clinical decisions.

As novice nurses enter the workforce, they are supported by their organizations in multiple ways. During the transition period, they are developing efficiencies that are important as they become advanced beginner nurses and then competent nurses. It is important for nurses to receive support in their journey to competency to gain efficiency while providing quality patient outcomes. This article explores opportunities to develop efficiencies as nurses enter practice. There are opportunities in personal support and with system support. Nurse leaders support novice nurses by facilitating proper professional experiences and proper system support.

Mental illness is one of the leading causes of disability in the United States. Delays in outpatient treatment result in visits to emergency rooms and unnecessary inpatient hospitalizations, which cause an increase in overall medical costs. Nurses come in contact with individuals who struggle with mental illness on a regular basis, and the profession must intervene. This article introduces the mental health outpatient nurses in interprofessional teams model that could have a positive impact on the quality and accessibility of care of outpatient services for individuals struggling with mental illness.

Faculty mentoring of undergraduate students is an essential and necessary component in helping students achieve exposure and success in cocurricular activities that they may not get in the classroom. It is through these cocurricular activities that faculty can expose students to the realms of various clinical activities, nursing research and education, and various service-related opportunities, such as tutoring and committee work. The intrinsic and extrinsic awards of watching your students succeed and grow into nursing leaders make mentoring worth it. This article outlines the benefits and difficulties experienced by 1 faculty member in his crusade to mentor undergraduate nursing students.

Sepsis is a deadly and costly condition, but effectively managing sepsis in the emergency department (ED) can help to improve patient outcomes. A key part of sepsis management is improving compliance with sepsis bundles, which can be challenging in the ED setting. Bedside nurses in the ED have a unique opportunity to facilitate early identification and treatment of patients with sepsis, which increases sepsis bundle compliance and improves patient outcomes. Interventions reviewed in this article can help to improve early identification and treatment, along with ways to standardize care, provide education, and implement feedback.

The Veterans Health Administration Home Based Primary Care (VHA-HBPC) program serves Veterans with complex, chronic conditions. Emergency management is a concern for VHA-HBPC programs. Geographic information system (GIS) mapping has been implemented for local program operations in 30 locations. An evaluation assessed GIS mapping as a tool in emergency management, including frontline nurses' and nurse leaders' experiences. Nurses' roles included making and using maps for preparedness and response. Maps provided valuable information, including locations of vulnerable patients (eg, ventilator dependent), community emergency resources, and environmental threats (eg, hurricane). Nurses' willingness to embrace this new technology and skill set was notable.

The release of a quality study by the Institute of Medicine in 2001 challenged health care providers to deliver safe, quality care. Research has focused on 2 primary categories of nursing characteristics: demographic data and emotional intelligence and personality traits. The research has shown a correlation between nursing characteristics and quality care and patient outcomes. Factors not considered in this article include hospital teaching status, type of unit, unit skill mix, hospital safety culture, and total nursing hours per patient day. These factors may contribute to quality of care and patient outcomes.

Development of clinical nurses in Magnet-designated organizations is enhanced through a commitment to shared governance principles, a relevant and visible professional practice model, and engagement of clinical nurses in shared decision making. Cultivating practice innovations and reward and recognition programs further assist to sustain this development and leads to growth of future leaders.

To meet the significant increase in the demand for home health care, retention of home health nurses is essential. Job satisfaction is the major determinant of retention. Assessment of satisfaction indicators is a useful method to inform a home health agency plan to improve job satisfaction of home health nurses. Satisfaction was assessed using a standardized instrument, the Home Healthcare Nurse Job Satisfaction scale. The outcomes of a quality improvement process informed the development of a retention plan strategy to help leaders retain this important nursing work force in home health.

NURSING CLINICS OF
NORTH AMERICA

FORTHCOMING ISSUES

June 2020
Orthopedic Nursing
Tandy Gabbert, *Editor*

September 2020
SexuallyTransmitted Infections
Courtney J. Pitts, *Editor*

December 2020
Complementary and Alternative Medicine,
Part I: Therapies
Stephen Krau, *Editor*

RECENT ISSUES

December 2019
Psychiatric Disorders
Rene Love, *Editor*

September 2019
Transitions of Care for Patients with
Neurological Diagnoses
Sonja E. Stutzman, *Editor*

June 2019
Infectious Diseases
Randolph F. R. Rasch, *Editor*

SERIES OF RELATED INTEREST

Critical Care Nursing Clinics of North America
https://www.ccnursing.theclinics.com/

THE CLINICS ARE AVAILABLE ONLINE!
Access your subscription at:
www.theclinics.com

Foreword

Is Emotional Intelligence an Important Trait for Nurse Managers and Leaders?

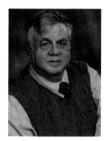

Stephen D. Krau, PhD, RN, CNE
Consulting Editor

It has been suggested by Tyczkowski and colleagues[1] that stress and lack of support for the role of nurse managers are among the reasons that less than 12.5% of nurses aspire to leadership roles. [1] They suggest that the trait of *resiliency* enables one to adapt to adversity, and tension is integral to an effective nurse manager and is a predictor of a manager's success. As health care becomes more complex and continues to evolve, the skills, knowledge, and behaviors of nurse managers must also evolve. This evolution is accompanied by an increase in stress among nurse managers. Emotional Intelligence (EI) is a means to enhance psychological resiliency to ameliorate stressors as high levels of EI have been shown to enhance transformational leadership style, which contributes to the provision and support of a positive and effective work environment.[2]

EI embodies the ability to identify and regulate one's own emotions as well as the emotions of others. The notion of EI includes the 3 following basic skills: (1) Emotional awareness, which is the ability to identify one's own emotions, while discriminating among variant emotions; (2) the ability to utilize those emotions in order to apply them to charges such as thinking and problem solving; and (3) the ability to manage those emotions, which includes regulating one's own emotions and helping others regulate their emotions. EI is sometimes referred to as "Emotional Quotient" (EQ), which holds wide interest and has been used in the interview processes of several well-known companies. The theory is that persons with higher levels of EI make better coworkers and/or make more effective leaders. In addition, EI is a skill that can be honed through training, journaling, and counseling. Persons with high levels of EI are conscious of their own emotional states and are also attuned to the emotions others experience. The ability to see how emotional sensitivity to emotional signals from

Nurs Clin N Am 55 (2020) xiii–xiv
https://doi.org/10.1016/j.cnur.2019.12.002
0029-6465/20/© 2019 Published by Elsevier Inc.

within and from the professional environment could make one a better leader. Although a gold standard for the measurement of EI has yet to be identified, there are many tools that have been developed to measure EI. One tool used to measure EQ is the *Bar-on EQ-I survey tool*, which has recently been used in a study by Tyczkowski and colleagues.[1]

One leadership style that is often considered desirable in the ever-changing health care milieu is *transformational leadership*. This form of leadership relates to resiliency among nurse leaders as well as those they manage. As attrition and burnout are common elements in many health care settings, there is evidence to suggest that transformational leadership is significantly related to increased satisfaction, increased staff well-being, decreased burnout, and decreased overall stress in staff nurses.[3] Transformational leadership is a leadership style in which nurse leaders encourage, inspire, and motivate nurses to innovate and create change that will help grow and structure the future success of the health care institution. The basis of transformational leadership includes individualized consideration, intellectual stimulation, inspirational motivation, and idealized influence. Whereas there are other styles of leadership, transformational leadership has particular implications for the ever-changing and stressful health care system. Numerous studies have shown a positive correlation among staff that works with leaders who have been identified as transformational leaders.[1] The study by Tycyzkowski and colleagues[1] shows results congruent to many studies that there is a "significant positive relationship between EI factors and transformational leadership style."[1(p.177)]

The results of the evidence related to EI and transformational leadership support the need to recruit, educate, and keep topmost performing leaders and managers in nursing. If not a part of the initial interview, EI assessment and development can be a part of the manager's career trajectory. Because EI can be learned, it would be worthwhile for health care systems to provide training and counseling to nursing leaders and managers as well as nurses who are potential nurse leaders.

Stephen D. Krau, PhD, RN, CNE
Vanderbilt University School of Nursing
6809 Highland Park Drive
Nashville, TN 37205, USA

E-mail address:
sdkrau@outlook.com

REFERENCES

1. Tyczkowski B, Vandenbouten C, Reilly J, et al. Emotional Intelligence (EI) and nursing leadership styles among nurse managers. Nurs Admin Q 2015;39(2): 172–80.
2. Barling J, Slater F, Kelloway K. Transformational leadership and emotional intelligence: an exploratory study. Leadersh Organ Dev J 2000;21:157–61.
3. Weberg D. Transformational leadership and staff retention: an evidence review with implications for healthcare systems. Nurs Admin Q 2010;34(3):246–58.

Preface

Nurses Leading Innovation

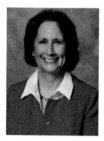

Kelly A. Wolgast, DNP, RN, FACHE, FAAN
Editor

Nurses in today's complex health care environment have the knowledge, skill, and ability to lead change through innovation at the point of care. With the demand for greater access, the delivery of health care is now expanded beyond the traditional hospital setting. The point of care is far ranging from a physical care setting to a virtual encounter using technology-supported communications between nurses and patients. In this issue of *Nursing Clinics of North America*, the focus is on sharing insights on how nurses are prepared as leaders to provide innovative care for our patients and to present thoughts on how the care environment can further support ongoing innovation by nurses.

The articles in this issue take us on a journey through innovation in various nursing care environments as well as present perspective on how leadership innovation is embedded in nursing education. As nurses, we strive to be the best patient advocates. Nursing students are educated to recognize vulnerable populations and to seek out sustainability solutions to help influence environmental change to support health and well-being. Nurses can and should be leaders in promoting population health through policy development and use of social media to educate stakeholders and extend and amplify messages in support of health care issues. Within the hospital setting, nurses are making a difference as unit champions to lead quality improvement projects, such as implementing effective bedside rounding and improving sepsis management with a bundle approach and feedback mechanisms. Nurses at the bedside can and are garnering leadership buy-in for innovations in how care is provided to improve the patient experience and outcomes. Nurses are also making important clinical decisions based on evidence-based knowledge and experience. We present important insights on how nurses use intuition, experience, information use, and environmental pattern recognition for decision making in support of quality care.

Leading innovation requires that nurses make good decisions about personal supports and that nurse managers advocate for strong system supports for nurses at

https://doi.org/10.1016/j.cnur.2019.12.001
0029-6465/20/© 2019 Published by Elsevier Inc.
nursing.theclinics.com

the point of care. It is vital for nurses to learn and grow in competence within a health care system that values and acknowledges nurses and nursing. There is need to understand that characteristics of nurses can impact quality of care. These characteristics include social skills, personality traits, and emotional intelligence. Mentoring of nurses professionally in practice and while the nurse is in their nursing education is vital to ensuring that we support the professional socialization of nurses throughout the education and career lifespan. Students provide us with their viewpoints, which are powerful to read.

Nurses are part of creative and innovative care initiatives in a variety of settings. One author presents a care model with nurses for patients in an outpatient behavioral health setting providing increased access for this needed health care. Another presents the application of quality improvement to assess the satisfaction and retention needs of home health nurses, a growing role in nursing. Nurses and partners in the Veterans Health Administration are applying state-of-the-art technology in geographic-information-system mapping to identify vulnerable Veterans Administration patients that may need a higher level of coordinated care during times of natural disaster or other emergencies. This technology also can be applied to identify staff that also may be impacted by the same emergency conditions. Colleagues in a Magnet-designated facility reinforce the importance of promoting an environment in which nurses are encouraged to develop clinically and to sustain practice innovations.

I am delighted to share this issue that clearly demonstrates the willingness of nurses at the point of care, no matter where that point of care may be, to be proactive to gather the necessary information, make critical decisions, communicate positive solutions, care for each other, and care deeply for patients and families, all while promoting the best possible care environment for all people everywhere.

Kelly A. Wolgast, DNP, RN, FACHE, FAAN
College of Nursing, The Pennsylvania State University
203B Nursing Sciences Building
University Park, PA 16802, USA

E-mail address:
kaw466@psu.edu

Creating a Generation of Sustainable Nurses
Sustainability Efforts in Nursing Education

Erin Kitt-Lewis, PhD, RN[a],*, Marianne Adam, PhD, RN, CRNP[b],
Peter Buckland, PhD[c], Darlene Clark, MS, RN[d],
Kristal Hockenberry, MSN, RN[e], Diane Jankura, MA[f],
Janet Knott, DNP, RN, CNE[g]

KEYWORDS

- Curriculum • Health • Nurse leaders • Nursing education • Sustainability

KEY POINTS

- Emerging nurse leaders are not adequately prepared to handle the pervasive health care problems and threats related to the changing environment.
- Sustainability is a new concept emerging in the discipline of nursing.
- The inclusion of environmental sustainability in nursing education is foundational if students are to become informed members, advocates, and emerging leaders of a broader health care team.
- Several strategies are outlined and discussed as an approach to implementing environmental sustainability in nursing education and cultivating a culture of sustainability as an example for emerging nurse leaders.
- Nursing faculty must advocate for and adopt education practices to prepare nurses to recognize vulnerable populations and advocate for successful changes to the environment.

INTRODUCTION

Emerging nurse leaders are not adequately prepared to handle the pervasive health care problems and threats related to the changing environment. In the current global

[a] College of Nursing, The Pennsylvania State University, 201 Nursing Sciences Building, University Park, PA 16802, USA; [b] College of Nursing, The Pennsylvania State University, 200 University Drive, Schuylkill Haven, PA 17972, USA; [c] Penn State's Sustainability Institute, Educational Theory and Policy, 102 Land and Water Building, University Park, PA 16802, USA; [d] College of Nursing, The Pennsylvania State University, 205B Nursing Sciences Building, University Park, PA 16802, USA; [e] College of Nursing, The Pennsylvania State University, 25 Nursing Sciences Building, University Park, PA 16802, USA; [f] College of Nursing, The Pennsylvania State University, 203 Nursing Sciences Building, State College, PA 16802, USA; [g] College of Nursing, The Pennsylvania State University, Penn State New Kensington, 3550 Seventh Street Road, New Kensington, PA 15068-1765, USA
* Corresponding author.
E-mail address: eak114@psu.edu

Nurs Clin N Am 55 (2020) 1–10
https://doi.org/10.1016/j.cnur.2019.10.001
0029-6465/20/© 2019 Elsevier Inc. All rights reserved.

environment, population health risks are increasing at alarming rates. Anthropogenic climate change already threatens human health and well-being through extreme weather events, wildfire, decreased air quality, stress, and food-borne, water-borne, and pest-borne diseases. It will continue to amplify existing health issues, especially for at-risk people and some communities of color.[1] In fact, 23% of global deaths and 26% of deaths among children under five are due to modifiable environmental factors, from chemical exposure, air and water pollution, and diseases found in the home, coming from transit, energy production, and others.[2] With a variety of increased health risks to people of all ages and socioeconomic backgrounds, it is necessary to educate and prepare nurses to recognize vulnerable populations and advocate for successful changes to the environment.[3,4] Many dangers to health are prevalent in the home and work environments, which increases the need for nurses to have a strong foundation in advocacy of health promotion, environmental health, and social justice.[5] Facing these challenges to the current health care systems, faculty must be prepared to educate the new generation of nurses on the connection between health and the environment. By addressing these issues proactively in nursing education, institutions will develop nurse leaders who are well positioned to improve the quality of patient outcomes as well as decreasing health care costs.

BACKGROUND

The concept of sustainability in nursing originated with Florence Nightingale. Nightingale's[7] environmental theory of nursing contains the core principle that nursing is the act of using the environment as a tool for enhancing the patient's recovery process,[6–8] and she states that, "Nature alone cures ... and what nursing has to do in either case, is to put the patient in the best condition for nature to act upon him."[7]

She thought that managing patients' surroundings to best meet the current needs of the patients would assist in the healing process.[6–8] Nightingale[7] thought that there were many natural elements that could assist with the restoration of health. She proposed that nursing was more than just emotionally caring for a patient, following doctors' orders, or meeting physical and nutritional needs. She advocated that a patient could, "unmake what God had made disease to be" with light, warmth, fresh air, quiet, and cleanliness in the surrounding environment.[7]

Nightingale's general beliefs have been integrated into modern-practice concepts, including those aspects of human health that are determined by the physical, chemical, biological, social, and psychological problems in the environment.[9] The American Nurses Association (ANA) Principles of Environmental Health for Nursing Practice with Implementation Strategies is a document whose purpose is to guide environmentally safe nursing care.[10,11] There are 10 principles included in this document, which encourage nurses to act in order to facilitate evidence-based practice by gaining a working understanding of how human health and environmental exposure are integrally connected.[10] Since Nightingale's tenure more than 100 years ago, mounting evidence shows the impact of climate change on social and environmental determinants of health (ie, clean and safe air and drinking water, sufficient food, and shelter), emphasizing the importance for nursing faculty to acknowledge the need to integrate these 10 principals into nursing education. For the last 10 years, there has been a call by the ANA to integrate this knowledge into basic nursing education and practice,[10] but little has been done.

The International Council of Nurses (ICN), the governing body of the ANA, also thinks that nurses and the nursing profession play a vital role in mitigating the negative impact on the environment of medical waste and the products used in health care.[3] In

2018, ICN asserted that climate change is the largest threat to global development and is also a threat to the progress made in public health over the past 50 years.[3] Therefore, there is a demand for nurses to be educated to deliver integrated models of evidence-based care to prevent or delay the progression of diseases related to climate change. In collaboration with the ICN, the World Health Organization (WHO) has mandated that nurses promote healthy environments.[9] Nurses have historically prided themselves on providing holistic care to patients and their communities, and the modern era is no exception. There is currently a movement started by nurses who are passionate about sustaining a healthy future by using ecocentric nursing (ie, earth-centered care, which includes the physical and natural environments and the systems that nurses work in).

Good health and well-being has now been recognized in the international system by the United Nations Agenda 2030: The Sustainable Development Goals. Goal 3 commits the international order to "ensure healthy lives and promote well-being for all at all ages."[10] Importantly, this goal is viewed as part of a holistic nexus of social, economic, environmental, governance, and partnership goals. For example, accomplishing goal 3 can only be achieved with consummate action in goal 6 (clean water and sanitation), a target of which commits to "[improving] water quality by reducing pollution, eliminating dumping and minimizing release of hazardous chemicals and materials, halving the proportion of untreated wastewater and substantially increasing recycling and safe reuse globally [by 2030]."[10] Other examples in educational, gender-related, energy-related, infrastructural, and climate-related goals have a direct bearing on human health. In addition, when pursued holistically across sectors, ecological benefits can accrue such that action on clean water and sanitation acts positively on targets and indicators under goal 14 (conserve and sustainably use the oceans, seas, and marine resources for sustainable development).[10]

Nursing educators are joining a global decades-old sustainability education and training movement that is gaining speed and momentum. In 1990, the University Leaders for a Sustainable Future, wrote the *Talloires Declaration*, which calls for the "stabilization of human population, adoption of environmentally sound industrial and agricultural technologies, reforestation, and ecological restoration"[12] and for universities to "initiate and support mobilization of internal and external resources so that their institutions respond to this urgent challenge."[12] In 1992, the Earth Summit brought environmental education, human rights, and human development together and called for broad and deep educational transformation to develop education, public awareness, and training toward sustainable development.[13] The United Nations continues to recognize and support education and training as critical to sustainable development, and explicitly mentions higher education as a critical sector in achieving Agenda 2030: The Sustainable Development Goals. Goal 4.B reads:

> By 2020, substantially expand globally the number of scholarships available to developing countries, in particular least developed countries, small island developing States and African countries, for enrolment [sic] in higher education, including vocational training and information and communications technology, technical, engineering and scientific programmes, in developed countries and other developing countries.[10]

In the United States, colleges and universities are working toward this goal through associations; the creation of sustainability offices, centers, and institutes; and through curricular integration in general education as well as across and inside disciplines.

Over the last several years, sustainability has made its way into many disciplinary degree programs across the United States. In 2017, the National Council for Science and the Environment reported that 872 higher education institutions host 2361 interdisciplinary environmental, sustainability, and energy degree programs.[14] Some of these programs have a health emphasis. For example, Macalester College offers a Bachelor of Arts in environmental studies with a specialization in community and global health.[14] These institutions also host 2222 disciplinary professional degree programs that integrate environment, sustainability, or energy.[14] Of those programs, 212 are in health disciplines.[14] These programs span arts; engineering; humanities; professional; policy; and biological, physical, and social sciences.

The Sustainability Tracking Assessment & Rating System (STARS) is a self-reporting framework for colleges and universities to measure their sustainability performance. This program was developed by the Association for the Advancement of Sustainability in Higher Education (AASHE) with the intention of engaging and recognizing communities and institutions for their sustainable efforts.[15] Through participating in STARS, institutions can earn points toward a STARS bronze, silver, gold, or platinum rating, or earn the STARS Reporter designation. Each seal represents significant sustainability leadership. In 2017, Penn State received a gold rating from STARS, which is an improvement from 2011 when Penn State received a STARS silver rating. According to Penn State's STARS report, several colleges (ie, colleges of agricultural sciences, arts and architecture, business, earth and mineral sciences, and health and human development) house degree programs, minors, or certificates with sustainability requirements and a small number of intercollege minors focus on sustainability. There are more than 350 courses dispersed across nearly every college, varying from general education to discipline-specific advanced courses. Penn State College of Nursing is currently engaged in curricular innovations that will create general education opportunities and will revise our 4-year undergraduate program. This endeavor will integrate a holistic understanding of sustainability using Agenda 2030 and 2 complementary sustainability competencies frameworks that emphasize systems thinking, temporal or futures thinking, ethical or normative literacy, interpersonal skills, strategic thinking, and creativity and imagination.[16]

Nursing Education and Sustainability

Nurse educators prepare nurses for an extensive variety of roles and responsibilities necessary to meet the health care needs of society. These nurses practice in all settings from public health to acute care across the country and the world. The inception of Standard 17: Environmental Health in the ANA scope of practice and the Institute of Medicine (IOM) report recommended the inclusion of environmental health in all levels of nursing education, which prompted a closer look into the nursing curriculum.[17] To incorporate the key dimensions necessary to provide a comprehensive curriculum around sustainable initiatives, competencies and educational strategies must be clearly defined and outlined.[18] Included in the curriculum should be critical content that addresses the environmental impacts of globalization, food insecurity and influences of the production processes, the effects of smoking and other environmental effects on the health of children, the proper use of resources and management of waste, and methods for health promotion.[18] Educational approaches, such as the participatory action research and problem-based learning, provide sound strategies for implementing environmental sustainability in the curriculum. Current nursing curriculum will need to be systematically assessed for content related to environmental health, and resources including educational opportunities for engagement need to be embedded to facilitate lifelong learning in environmental health. Interprofessional educational opportunities with a variety of academic disciplines within and outside health care bring a variety of perspectives to environmental health topics that strengthen all programs.

Educating the Next Generation of Nurses

At least 5 generations of nurses coexist in the workplace; each of these generations has unique styles and preferences.[19] Although each of the 5 generations of nurses who work in health care is unique, a common nexus is that all nurses attend to patients who have been diagnosed with a chronic disease that was caused by an environmental pollutant. Nurses from all generations embrace the central goals of understanding and preventing chronic diseases.

The information age, interlinked with technology, has enabled the estimated 19 million nurses worldwide to connect and to build alliances and organizational platforms for health care providers to work collaboratively. For this reason, nurses are empowered to promote and advocate for healthy environments, plus practice in an environmentally safe and healthy manner.[19] This generation of nursing students, like their predecessors, is eager to get involved. At Penn State, for example, students served on the Penn State College of Nursing Sustainability Committee, performed a needs assessment related to environmental sustainability, and developed an activity to specifically address a priority need, partnering with student organizations on other campuses to enhance the Lion Pantry (campus food bank) for students experiencing food insecurity.

COLLEGE OF NURSING SUSTAINABILITY INITIATIVES

Beginning in 2015 and as part of their strategic plan, the Penn State College of Nursing formalized their sustainability initiatives. While each initiative will be discussed in detail below, a timeline is provided to outline these efforts (**Fig. 1**). The first initiative was to create a sustainability task force (ie, Sustainability Committee). The committee was created in 2015 and charged with launching new initiatives that promote stewardship of material resources. The committee members include faculty, staff, and students from 3 campuses. Although the committee is only required to meet quarterly, monthly

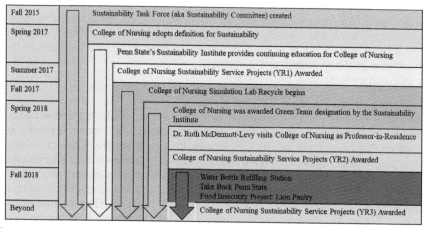

Fig. 1. College of nursing sustainability initiative timeline. YR, year.

meetings were necessary to monitor ongoing initiatives. In addition, committee members have created a strong collaboration with Penn State's Sustainability Institute. A key member of that group and coauthor of this article, Peter Buckland, agreed to partner with us and regularly attends the College of Nursing Sustainability Committee meetings.

The College of Nursing defines sustainability as the simultaneous pursuit of human health and happiness, environmental quality, and economic well-being for current and future generations and created a path to engage students and faculty together in funded sustainability service projects. This definition was created by the College of Nursing with collaboration from the broader Penn State community and the Sustainability Institute and adopted by the College of Nursing in 2017.

The service project initiative began after representatives from the Sustainability Institute provided a continuing education program at our spring faculty meeting in 2017. The College of Nursing's initial sustainability initiative began with the award of a grant proposal from the Sustainability Institute to implement a clean medical waste recycling program in the nursing simulation laboratory. Historically, the materials used in the simulation laboratory were disposed of in the regular trash or medical waste receptacles. Approximately 80% of the products used in the simulation laboratory are now recycled, composted, or reused. Bins specifically designated with recycling/composting signage are present in pods throughout the simulation laboratory spaces. Students watch a 5-minute video clip that clearly defines the appropriate placement of recyclable products. A Green Team designation was awarded from the Sustainability Institute for this initiative.

In March 2018, faculty participated in continuing education programs addressing sustainability issues and ideas with a professor in residence, Dr Ruth McDermott-Levy, from Villanova University. Dr McDermott-Levy spent a week with the College of Nursing and the wider Penn State community visiting classes in sustainability and leadership; meeting with faculty, undergraduate students, and graduate students in the Architecture and Landscape Architecture programs; meeting staff from the Sustainability Institute and Institutes of Energy and the Environment; and presenting to the public on issues such as global health, the impacts of fracking, climate change, and the United Nations Sustainable Development Goals.

Sustainability Service Projects

The College of Nursing grant also designated funds to support sustainability initiatives. Proposals are accepted annually and vetted through the Sustainability Committee, and the Dean of the College of Nursing selects the projects to be implemented. One key criterion is the inclusion and participation of students on the project. To date the following projects have been funded.

Water bottle refilling station

Sustainable Filtered Water Alternatives: Local to Global Effects is a project that is focused on increasing awareness of the devastating effects of disposable plastic water bottles. The goal of this project is to educate those who use the nursing simulation laboratory on the benefits of using the filtered water bottle station to refill their reusable bottles. An educational poster above the refill station provides current facts on the numerous benefits of filtered water, reusable bottles, and how students can become more involved in sustainability at Penn State. The team working on this project included 2 nursing students and 1 nursing faculty member. This project was completed in the spring 2019 semester.

Take back Penn state

Take Back Penn State is an initiative to deliver evidence-based education to the university community on the safe and responsible disposable of expired and unwanted medications. The goal of the project is 2-fold: to involve undergraduate and graduate students in raising awareness about the potential threats this problem has to the community, and to better understand the problem of unwanted/expired medications on the Penn State community. This project was inspired by the Department of Drug Enforcement Administration National Prescription Take Back Program. The Take Back Penn State team includes 1 graduate student, 3 undergraduate students, an instructional designer, a librarian, a police officer, and 2 nursing faculty members. The intended outcomes are to create evidence-based educational modules/presentations, develop a Web site, and educate students (n = 500) and employees (n = 500). Before the education initiative, a Qualtrics survey will be sent to all campus e-mail recipients asking employees and students about their medication disposal behaviors and knowledge. The educational program will take place over the fall semester. The same survey will be sent out at the end of the semester and compared with the previous survey.

Food insecurity project

The Penn State Lion Pantry was started several years before the College of Nursing initiatives to help with food insecurities of college students at the Behrend campus within the larger university system. As part of a clinical assignment in a core nursing course, nursing students could select the Lion Pantry project as their undergraduate community health course service-learning project. In 2018, 4 students selected the Lion Pantry project and collaborated with the campus AmeriCorps VISTA (Volunteers in Service to America) Food Security Liaison and a commonwealth campus student organization committed to helping the Lion Pantry as part of this service-learning project. Initially, the students conducted a needs assessment and developed an activity specifically to address priority needs. As a result of the assessment and needs prioritization assignment, the service activity involved fundraising to sustain the program and market the new program on the Behrend campus. In addition, it is a course requirement that each student enrolled in the course spend at least 10 hours working with the Lion Pantry, which is beyond the time designated to conduct the assessment and prioritization activity.

Curriculum Development Integrating Sustainability

Convinced that human health is greatly affected by environmental factors, the Sustainability Committee asked the key member from the Sustainability Institute to examine the undergraduate nursing curriculum by reviewing each course syllabus, objectives, and outcomes. The purpose of this curriculum review was to identify areas where sustainability issues are already being addressed and to offer suggestions for further enhancement without compromising the essentials of the curriculum. As the committee discussed the sustainability issues that were areas of strength and the potential for future integration into the curriculum, the committee thought that a stand-alone course could be created that would emphasize this interrelatedness. The committee is currently developing a 3-credit elective (45 semester hours) that will encourage students to actively engage in examining their world and the daily choices they make that could have an impact on their own health or the health of others. The goal for this course is to become part of the general education curriculum, cross-listed as a natural science and health course open to students of all majors, but with specific emphasis on those who will soon be leaders in science, food production, and engineering, as well as those who will become the teachers and providers of health care.

DISCUSSION

Opportunities to incorporate sustainability initiatives within the nursing courses and curriculum are shown by the Penn State College of Nursing activities, including the sustainability service projects, the curriculum review, and course development. Nursing faculty can take several approaches to sustainability content incorporation. Theoretic or philosophic foundation may guide this incorporation. Similar to this College of Nursing, a curriculum review may clearly identify content currently integrated into courses, as well as uncover areas where additional content could be integrated into the current curriculum. Classroom or laboratory activities focused on natural disasters are a suggested starting point. The activity could include review of predisaster variables through disaster recovery and postdisaster planning, including the roles of the nurse.[20] Allotting for a debriefing phase could launch discussions to include ethics, policy, and advocacy. A similar approach could be used when discussing biological events such as the Ebola outbreak[21] or current measles outbreak.[22] A different approach and more global approach is to incorporate the sustainable development goals as outlined by the United Nations in targeted courses or threaded throughout the curriculum.[23] No matter the approach for implementation, advocating for the adoption of sustainable initiatives in the curricula will enhance nursing education. Future goals include developing an interdisciplinary minor in sustainability.

Beyond the curriculum, fostering a culture that embraces sustainability practices in the academic setting will model behaviors that emphasize the importance of being a responsible global citizen, consumer, and clinician. A consistent finding supports the notion that social and physical contextual factors strongly influence human behavior when thinking about sustainability practices.[24] Creating a physical and social environment that cultivates positive sustainable practices will show the expectation early in their career trajectory. Ultimately such behavioral practices would be sustained for the duration of their careers, further influencing the next generation of nurses and beyond.

Specifically, nursing faculty play an important role in preparing the students to be competent clinicians and emerging leaders in health care. Nursing students think that being a positive role model is an essential characteristic of nursing faculty. Students' expectations are that faculty should show the same qualities that the students are being asked to emulate.[25] Faculty members who work side by side with nursing students have a responsibility to influence students' global perspectives in clinical practices and beyond. Nursing faculty can leverage this influence to promote practices focused on sustainable initiatives. Establishing a committee focused on strategic planning to enhance sustainability efforts in the college/department could prove to be an efficient and effective approach to cultivating current and future nurse leaders to collectively improve the quality of health for all. Raising awareness at an individual, departmental/college, and university level is necessary for establishing interest, motivation, and buy-in to sustainability efforts. An initial first step may be a review of college/department consumption practices to inform policy related to recycling, office and clinical laboratory supplies, and the environment. Over the course of the nursing program, students should be expected to adopt these practices during all classroom and clinical experiences.

Nurses, who dedicate their professional lives to making the lives of others and their communities better, have a natural fit with sustainability. Despite Nightingale's early introduction of the concept of the relationship to health and the environment, sustainability is a new concept emerging in nursing.[26] It is a multifaceted concept embedded within a systems framework and influenced by international, national, and local factors.[16,27] Translating this concept into nursing education is necessary to address modern issues that face health care and nurses but could prove challenging. However, nursing education is inherently forward looking and considers critical issues that students are likely to encounter over the course of their professional careers. Given the current global environment, and as population health risks continue to increase at staggering rates, the inclusion of environmental sustainability in nursing education is foundational if students are to become informed members of a broader health care team, advocates for conscientious and ethical resource use, and contributors to improved patient outcomes. Nursing faculty must advocate for and adopt education practices to educate and prepare nurses to recognize vulnerable populations and advocate for successful changes to the environment.

DISCLOSURE

The authors have no commercial or financial conflicts of interest. Funding was received from the Sustainability Institute at Penn State for the Nursing Simulation Laboratory Recycling of Medical Waste and Organic Composting Program. Funding was received from the Penn State College of Nursing for the 3 sustainability projects: Take Back Penn State, Lion Pantry, and Sustainable Filtered Water Alternatives: Local to Global Effects.

REFERENCES

1. Hess JJ, Eidson M, Tlumak JE, et al. An evidence-based public health approach to climate change adaptation. Environ Health Perspect 2014;122:1177–86.
2. Prüss-Ustün A, Wolf J, Corvalán C, et al. Diseases due to unhealthy environments: an updated estimate of the global burden of disease attributable to environmental determinants of health. J Public Health (Oxf) 2016;39(3):464–75.
3. International Council of Nurses. Position statement: nurses, climate change and health 2018. Available at: https://www.icn.ch/sites/default/files/inline-files/PS_E_Nurses_climate%20change_health.pdf. Accessed May 1, 2019.
4. Leffers J, Levy RM, Nicholas PK, et al. Mandate for the nursing profession to address climate change through nursing education. J Nurs Scholarsh 2017; 49(6):679–87.
5. Polivka BJ, Chaudry RV. A scoping review of environmental health nursing research. Public Health Nurs 2018;35(1):10–7.
6. Selanders LC. The power of environmental adaptation: florence Nightingale's original theory for nursing practice. J Holist Nurs 2010;28(1):81–8.
7. Nightingale F. Notes on nursing: what it is, and what it is not. New York: Barnes and Noble Publishing, Inc.; 2003 (originally published in 1860).
8. Hegge M. Nightingale's environmental theory. Nurs Sci Q 2013;26(3):211–9. https://doi.org/10.1177/0894318413489255. Available at:Accessed March 1, 2019.
9. World Health Organization. World health statistics 2016: monitoring health for the SDGs sustainable development goals. Geneva (Switzerland): World Health Organization; 2016.
10. American Nurses Association (ANA). American nurses association principles of environmental health for nursing practice with implementation strategies. Silver Springs (MD): American Nurses Association; 2007. Available at: http://ojin.nursingworld.org/MainMenuCategories/WorkplaceSafety/Healthy-Nurse/ANAs PrinciplesofEnvironmentalHealthforNursingPractice.pd. Accessed March 1, 2019.

11. United Nations sustainable development goals knowledge platform. Goal 4: quality education: targets and Indicators. Available at: https://sustainabledevelopment. un.org/sdg4. Accessed May, 2019.

12. University Leaders for a Sustainable Future. The talloires declaration 1990. Available at: http://www.ulsf.org/programs_talloires.html. Accessed March 1, 2019.

13. United Nations Commission on Sustainable Development. Agenda 21. 1992. Available at: http://sustainabledevelopment.un.org/content/documents/Agenda21.pdf. Accessed March 1, 2019.

14. Vincent S, Rao S, Fu Q, et al. Scope of interdisciplinary environmental, sustainability, and energy baccalaureate and graduate education in the United States. Washington, DC: National Council for Science and the Environment; 2017.

15. Association for the Advancement of Sustainability in Higher Education (AASHE). The sustainability tracking, assessment & rating systems 2019. Available at: https://www.aashe.org/. Accessed March 1, 2019.

16. Engle E, Barsom S, Vandenbergh L, et al. Developing framework for sustainability meta-competencies. Int J High Educ Sust 2017;1(4):285–303.

17. American Nurses Association (ANA). Nursing: scope and standards of practice. 3rd.edition. Silver Spring (MD): Nursesbooks.org; 2015.

18. Álvarez-Nieto C, López-Medina IM, Abad ML, et al. Curriculum nurse and strategies training on environmental sustainability and climate change. Global Nursing 2017;16(3):665–78.

19. Knight R. Managing people from five generations. Harv Bus Rev 2014;25(9):1–7.

20. Blais KK, Hayes JS. Professional nursing practice: concepts and perspectives. 7th edition. Boston: Pearson; 2016.

21. Centers for Disease Control and Prevention (CDC) Foundation. 2018 Ebola outbreak. 2019. Available at: https://www.cdcfoundation.org/2018-ebola-outbreak. Accessed May 1, 2019.

22. Centers for Disease Control and Prevention (CDC). Measles cases and outbreaks 2019. Available at: https://www.cdc.gov/measles/cases-outbreaks.html. Accessed May 1, 2019.

23. United Nations. Sustainable development goals. Available at: https://www.un.org/ sustainabledevelopment/sustainable-development-goals/. Accessed March 1, 2019.

24. Arbuthnott KD. Education for sustainable development beyond attitude change. Int J Sust Higher Ed 2009;10(2):152–63.

25. Niederriter JE, Eyth D, Thoman J. Nursing students' perceptions on characteristics of an effective clinical instructor. SAGE Open Nurs 2017;3. 2377960816685571.

26. Collins E, Ross J, Crawley J, et al. An undergraduate educational model for developing sustainable nursing practice: a New Zealand perspective. Nurse Educ Today 2018;61:264–8.

27. Wiek A, Withycombe L, Redman CL. Key competencies in sustainability: a reference framework for academic program development. Sustain Sci 2011;6(2): 203–18.

Promoting Population Health

Nurse Advocacy, Policy Making, and Use of Media

Carole R. Myers, PhD, RN

KEYWORDS

• Nurse advocacy • Policy making • Media engagement • Population health

KEY POINTS

- Nurses' engagement in policy making and advocacy extends the caring ethos of the nursing profession and is particularly relevant and important in promoting population health.
- A population perspective and an expanded complement of strategies and tools are necessary to improve health and health care beyond the bedside and individual patient encounter.
- Nurses should actively engage in evidence-based policy making by identifying problems, producing and translating evidence, evaluating public policies and programs, and advocating for needed changes.
- Media can be used to effectively highlight health and health care problems amenable to public policy solutions, educate stakeholders, and promote policy change.

INTRODUCTION

Nurses' engagement in policy making and advocacy extends the caring ethos of the nursing profession and is particularly relevant and important in promoting population health. It is incumbent upon nurses to use a population perspective and an expanded complement of strategies and tools to improve health and health care beyond the bedside and individual patient encounter. Nurses can be inspired to address contemporary and future challenges by reflecting on the works of nursing heroines, such as Lillian Wald, Dorothea Dix, and Florence Nightingale. These historical leaders embraced and modeled the delivery of population-based health care and nursing advocacy, and policy making. Contemporary nurses can use various forms of media

University of Tennessee, College of Nursing, 1200 Volunteer Boulevard. Knoxville, TN 37916, USA
E-mail address: cmyers9@utk.edu
Twitter: @TNPolicyNurse (C.R.M.)

Nurs Clin N Am 55 (2020) 11–20
https://doi.org/10.1016/j.cnur.2019.11.001
0029-6465/20/
© 2019 Elsevier Inc. All rights reserved.

to support policy engagement and advocate for needed changes to improve population health.

Contextual Influences

Despite spending almost 45% more on health care as a percentage of the gross domestic product than the next closest country among 10 other high-income countries, the United States has poorer health outcomes and is ranked last in health care system performance among the comparator countries.[1] Unacceptable disparities exist among certain populations, and the United States does not have guaranteed universal coverage for health care. There are numerous measures, such as all-cause mortality, premature death, death amenable to health care, and disease burden, whereby US performance is improving, but improvements are slower than those of other countries, and consequently, the gap between the United States and these countries is growing.[2]

A Call for Transformation

The *Future of Nursing* report included a set of recommendations to better prepare and position the nursing workforce to meet increasing and diverse societal needs and advance nurses' contributions as an essential component of the health care workforce and leaders in improving health and health care.[3] The capacity-building efforts that emanated from the *Future of Nursing* recommendations were largely successful.[4] These efforts were necessary but insufficient to meet the most important need, which is moving the needle on improving health outcomes and reducing disparities. These 2 aims are the focus of the *Future of Nursing 2020 to 2030* initiative.[5] This initiative aims to prompt significant change by moving beyond capacity-building; enhancing infrastructure; and the inclusion of nurses as key leaders in health promotion, health care delivery, and policy making. Significant and sustainable change requires a population perspective and an emphasis on the societal and environmental impediments to the attainment of the best possible health for all individuals and communities. The type of deep change needed requires systematic changes that are most commonly accomplished in the policy arena.

Nurses have a rich historical legacy of championing changes needed to improve health and health care. This legacy provides a good foundation for responding to contemporary challenges and paving the way for a better future. However, the profession is at critical nexus where purpose and roles related to the delivery of care and services, advocacy, and policy making must be reconceptualized. The ensuing discussion focuses on the need to pivot to a population health perspective and a new emphasis and definition of nursing roles related to advocacy and policy making in advancing population health. If you believe the adages that past behaviors are the best predictor of future behaviors or success breeds success, the outlook is good for nursing meeting challenges and seeing challenges as opportunities.

Population Health

Population health is "an approach to health that aims to improve the health of an entire population and to reduce health inequities among population groups. In order to reach the objectives, it looks at and acts upon the broad range of factors and conditions that have a strong influence on our health."[6] Defining characteristics of population health center on creating conditions in which individuals and families can be healthy by focusing on wellness, prevention, and health promotion; upstream or root causes of health problems; addressing the social, environmental, and other factors that influence health; and working with a broad complement of stakeholders to improve health.[7,8] The 2 primary aims of population health are to use evidence-based practice to (1) improve health outcomes and (2) reduce disparities.

Health disparities are differences or inequalities in health status or outcomes between people and populations.[9] Health disparities impose a burden on affected individuals and groups and are manifested by poor health, premature mortality, and morbidity. If a health disparity is attributable to a difference that is unnecessary and avoidable, it is viewed as unjust.[10] Nurses' involvement in policy making and advocacy is frequently directed at reducing disparities.

The *County Health Ranking Model* is a useful depiction of the many factors that impact population health and must be addressed to improve outcomes.[11] The model focuses on modifiable determinants. The model shows social and economic factors, including education, employment, income, family and social support, and community safety contributing 40% toward the 2 outcome measures, length, and quality of life. Health behaviors (eg, tobacco use, diet and exercise, alcohol and drug use, and sexual activity) contribute 30%; clinical care (access to and quality of care) weighs in at 20%, and the physical environment (air and water quality and housing and transit) accounts for 10%.

Individual care focuses on treatment of specific diseases and conditions by dealing primarily with medical and biological health determinants and downstream symptoms within the health care sector. In contrast, population health prioritizes wellness, prevention, and health promotion among entire populations by addressing social and other upstream determinants and relies on partnerships between health and other sectors to be successful.[12]

Many of the past nursing heroines provided population-based health care. A classic example is Lillian Wald, often called the mother of public health nursing, who worked among Eastern European immigrants of the Lower East Side of New York beginning in the late 1800s to improve living and working conditions and to provide community-based care. Wald promoted school-based nursing. Another heroine is Dorothea Dix, who advocated for humane treatment of indigent people and prisoners with mental illness. Last, Florence Nightingale focused on improving environmental conditions and care delivered to soldiers wounded during the Crimean War. Nightingale also embraced evidence-based practice long before the term was coined and widely used.

As nurses migrated from community-based practice settings in the early to mid-1900s to hospitals, their focus shifted from care of populations and health promotion to care of the individual and treatment of illness. The shift from a community focus to a hospital focus had a significant impact on nurse advocacy and policy making.

Social conditions and the environment significantly shape health status and outcomes. Addressing social and environmental deficiencies that impeded attainment of maximal health status is best accomplished by policy changes. That is precisely the reason improving population health requires effective nurse advocacy and involvement in policy making.

Nurse Advocacy

A basic definition of advocacy is the pleading the cause of another or defending a cause or proposal.[13] To advocate means to plead for, uphold, support, advance, further, defend, or propose. A richer definition and understanding of nurse advocacy can be gleaned from Fowler's work.[14] Fowler identified 4 advocate roles for nurses, including the nurse as (1) protector of rights, (2) preserver of values, (3) defender of personhood, and (4) champion of social justice. Protecting rights reflects a legalistic understanding of advocacy, and it is the most common manifestation of nurse advocacy. In this model, the nurse intercedes on behalf of clients, usually individual clients.

When a nurse acts to preserve values, the nurse advocate empowers individuals and assists clients who are incapable of participating in health care decision making to preserve client values and autonomy. As a defender of personhood, the nurse advocate focuses on human rights and common human needs. Doing this is the most broad and demanding form of nurse advocacy.

The core mission of the nursing profession is promoting health. Advocacy (and policy making) is essential to this mission.[15] Nurses have long advocated for patients at the individual level.[16] Advocacy directs at the individual level alone is not enough. Nurses need to advocate for systematic change, inclusive of the many factors that interact to determine health, if they are to foster a *Culture of Health* whereby individuals, populations, and communities have the opportunities needed to thrive.[17] Furthermore, a profession that establishes a relationship with clients, based on a social contract, such as nursing, is morally obligated to uphold justice within its domain.[18–21]

Select nurse advocates involved in health policy were interviewed by Gebbie and colleagues.[15] The following 3 key themes emerged from the interviews: participants confirm that there is an inextricable link between the disciplinary focus of the nursing profession and the leaders' activism; nursing knowledge and skills translate well in the policy arena and can be applied successfully to advance a nursing agenda for change; and nurses have the potential to be major policy players. However, they also mentioned that the power of nurses has not been fully unleashed or sufficiently sustained.

An informal profile of nurse leaders known to the author and the path that led them to being active in the policy arena reveal an important point about seizing opportunities that was also discussed by Gebbie and colleagues.[15] Nurses need to respond to opportunities as they are presented and engage in policy making, not necessarily wait for a specific, hoped-for opportunity. Opportunities necessitating a response include facing an obstacle in the workplace; government action or inaction; or ineffective action, including no action, among professional or community organizations. Other opportunities also include being recruited, encouraged, and/or mentored by someone associated with advocacy and policy making.

Karen Daley, past president of the American Nurses Association, frequently relates her advocacy awakening and involvement in policy making to working in an Emergency Department, sustaining a needle stick, and consequently being seropositive for the hepatitis C and the human immunodeficiency viruses.[22] The author previously was involved with another Emergency Department nurse who was instrumental in advancing a workplace violence bill in Tennessee to better protect nurses. It took several years and required overcoming major resistance to pass a bill that afforded nurses assaulted in the workplace the same protections conferred to police officers and sports referees attacked during the course of their work. The tide turned when credible, federal statistics about the high rate of assaults and the sequelae, including direct and indirect costs associated with injuries and disabilities, lost work time, and the human toll, were presented and discussed with key state legislators.

Another exemplary nurse leader and colleague is Robin Cogan. She is motivated by her experiences as a school nurse for a marginalized community in New Jersey and the dubious distinction of having 2 family members involved in a mass shooting. Cogan is a nationally recognized advocate for the value of school nurses, placing at least 1 nurse in every school, and policies rooted in evidence and designed to reduce the epidemic of gun violence in the United States.

Melanie Rogers, a public health nurse from Colorado, could not abide by the contradiction of promoting evidence-based practice when so many practicing nurses do not have access to databases and key sources needed for evidence-based practice. She started a successful Twitter campaign, using the phrase #NoJournalsNoEBP, to encourage academic and other organizations to provide needed access for nurses.

The author is recognized for her long-term promotion of full-practice authority for advanced practice registered nurses in Tennessee as a way to improve access to high-quality, cost-effective primary care, particularly in rural areas. Her engagement began almost 40 years ago as the owner and operator of a rural primary care clinic in the community where she lived. As a PhD-prepared researcher and faculty member, the author has added a focus on the disparities seen among rural populations to the work she does. Besides being an advocate and engaging in policy making, the author conducts research and evaluations that have the potential to complement her activism.

Policy Making: The Nurses' Roles

Public policy is a government's response to a societal problem. Policy making is essentially a decision-making process that occurs in a political environment. Policy making provides for the allocation of scarce resources in a politically charged, highly competitive environment. Involvement in policy making offers nurses an opportunity to influence social and other programs that have a profound impact on health and health care.

Legislation is only 1 aspect of policy making. Nurses need to work with various governmental institutions and actors to have maximal impact.[23] Nurses need to be involved throughout the policy-making cycle and pay attention to critical and sometimes neglected processes, including rulemaking and other regulatory aspects of policy, policy and program evaluation, and policy modification. Longest[24] considers policy making to have 3 steps: Policy formulation, implementation, and modification. Alternative depictions of the policy-making cycle include problem identification of definition, agenda setting, and policy formulation, adoption, and evaluation as separate steps. Nurses can contribute to policy making in a variety of specific ways, including identifying problems, producing and translating evidence to support policy choices, evaluating public policies and programs, and leading and participating in grassroots and professional advocacy.[16]

Nurses can promote evidence-based policy that is responsive to impacted individuals and populations. Nurses have an important understanding of the human aspects and impacts of proposed and existing policies. Nurses can offer insight regarding the policy consequences, intended and unintended.[23]

The *Future of Nursing* report includes a classic quote, "Nurses must see policy as something they can shape, rather than something that happens to them."[3(p8)] Unfortunately, too many nurses are reluctant to get involved in policy making. Results from a survey included in the *Future of Nursing* report reflect a troubling contradiction. Opinion leaders, including government officials; insurance, pharmaceutical, and health care company executives; and physicians, indicated how much influence nurses *would* have during debates about national health reform and the Affordable Care Act and how much influence they *should* have based on their professional position.

Predictions included in the *Future of Nursing*[3] report regarding how much influence nurses would have in national reform deliberations leading up to the passage of the Affordable Care Act fell far short of the influence respondents thought nurses should have. It is interesting to note that for major topics of concern, including medical errors and quality of care, an overwhelming number of opinion leaders, 90.4% and 88.9%, respectively, indicated nurses should be major players. The gap between what nurses should do and what they actually do represents a major opportunity for professional improvement.

Using Media

An important strategy for amplifying messages about societal problems amenable to public policy, educating stakeholders, bringing diverse people together for common purpose, and promoting change is the strategic use of traditional and social media. Media refer collectively to various forms of mass communication, including publishing, broadcasting, and the Internet.[25,26] Media are used to share news, entertain, educate, and for promotion.[25]

Nurses are persistently underrepresented in the media, both as sources and as subjects. The poor showing of nurses is illustrated in the 2 Woodhull studies, one conducted in 1997 (STTI [Sigma Theta Tau International]) and a 2018 follow-up study.[27] In both studies, nurses were absent from most stories despite the relevancy of a nursing perspective to the story (**Table 1**).

One conclusion of the study investigators is that because nursing is predominantly a female profession, the general underrepresentation of women is undoubtedly a factor (**Table 2**).

The lack of regard for nurses' positions and/or insight was evident in interviews with 10 journalists.[28] During interviews, journalists revealed they have to justify using nurses as sources to their editors, because nurses are not viewed as experts or key leaders, and, when contacted, organizations do not promote nurses as sources or subjects.

What are some of the strategies nurses can use to improve their media presence to enhance education and increase awareness on issues related to health and health care and advocate for needed policy and other changes? First and foremost, nurses need to use media and other communication strategies to effect change. The foundation of media and communication efforts is the art of messaging. Nurse messengers need to broadcast definitions of problems that need to be addressed, articulate definite positions about needed changes, and end with specific calls to action for individuals, populations, other nurses, and policymakers.

Nurses can respond to news items, offer a nursing perspective on a topic, and suggest individual, population, and societal responses. Options include writing letters to the editor in response to news item or authoring an op-ed to share expertise and propose solutions to specific problems, and offering to serve as a resource for print, radio, and television journalists and other media representatives. In doing any of these things, nurses should rely on a careful and proactive assessment and statement of the problem they are addressing, their commitment to improving health and health care, and a clear, professional articulation of what needs to be done, by who, and

Table 1 Key findings from 1997 and 2018 Woodhull studies		
Nurses	**1997**	**2018**
Percent quotes in newspapers	4	2
Percent quotes in weekly and industry publications	1	
Percent of time mentioned in article	14	13
Percent of time identified in photographs	0	4

Data from Mason DJ, Nixon L, Glickstein B, et al. The Woodhull study revisited: Nurses' representation in health news media 20 years later. J Nurs Scholarsh. 2018;50(6):695-704. https://doi.org/10.1111/jnu.12429 and Sigma Theta Tau International. Woodhull Study on Nursing and the Media: Health care's invisible partner. Final Report. Available at: https://sigma.nursingrepository.org/bitstream/handle/10755/624124/WoodhullReport1997.pdf?sequence=1&isAllowed=y. Accessed June 3, 2019.

Table 2
Nurses' representation in health news media

Nurse Inclusion	2018, Women, %	2018, Men, %
Quoted	34	65
Included in images	28	72

Data from Mason DJ, Nixon L, Glickstein B, Han S, Westphaln K, Carter L. The Woodhull study revisited: Nurses' representation in health news media 20 years later. *J Nurs Scholarsh.* 2018;50(6):695-704. https://doi.org/10.1111/jnu.12429.

when. **Table 3** shows a sampling of media types that nurses can use to promote change.

Why nurses? Nurses are well educated and have specialized expertise on major topics of broad interest. Nurses are trusted by the public and recognized as major health care players. Nurses can speak to the joys and sorrows of the human experience.

Nurses, and women in general, are underrepresented in the media despite the crucial role they have in promoting health and providing care to individuals, families, and communities. Nurses are cognizant of the problems encountered by people and groups of people in the pursuit of health and well-being and receiving health care and public health services.

It is also known that media are a powerful tool for educating, connecting, and organizing people for change. The ascendancy of social media is particularly noteworthy. Social media is a great equalizer. It is used by a broad spectrum of people from everyday citizens, celebrities, policy makers, scholars, and other leaders. Social media have fueled major contemporary social movements, including the prodemocracy

Table 3
Sampling of media types

Type of Media	Description	Uses
Letter to an editor (LTE)	Letter submitted to a publication by a reader; reaction or opinion about recent article, op-ed, or editorial. Generally short (250 words or less) and timely	Share professional and/or personal perspective in response to a recent news item or issue
Op-ed	Commentary with well-defined point-of-view on controversial, new, or current topic. Written by external contributors ("experts"). Longer than LTE; generally 750–1200 words	Highlight a specific problem, propose a specific action, and issue a call to action
Twitter	Real-time online social platform	Used to connect people, share news and other information, educate, and promote idea
Interviews (radio and television)	Discussion between a moderator or interviewers and respondents; can be live or prerecorded for broadcast on radio or television	Present and discuss information

protest dubbed the Arab Spring, the initial Women's March, and subsequent activities that aim to unite diverse women for transformative change, and the March for Our Lives movement that originated at Stoneman Douglas High School in Parkland, Florida following a tragic mass shooting at the school on February 14, 2018.

Robin Cogan, Melanie Rogers, and the author are skilled and active Twitter users; their Twitter handles are @RobinCogan, @MRogersRN, and @TNPolicy-Nurse. There are many other nurse Twitter aficionados. The hashtag #NursesWhoT-weet is gaining traction. Nurse Tweeters have been able to curate information related to their topics of interest, connect and collaborate with other stakeholders, and cultivate new ideas, such as seen in the Twitter hashtag, #NoJournalsNoEBP, created by Melanie Rogers.

SUMMARY

Transformative change is needed to improve health and health care in the United States. The barriers to improved health and the delivery of health care services originate in deeply rooted social and environmental deficiencies that must be acknowledged and addressed. Just as there is no single root cause of problems, there is no single solution to the problems. Nurses with a population perspective who are skilled and engaged in advocacy, policy making and media are essential for increasing the value of health care in the United States and in creating conditions whereby individuals and communities can thrive for the purpose of better health.

DISCLOSURE

No disclosures.

REFERENCES

1. Schneider EC, Sarnak DO, Squires D, et al. Mirror, mirror 2017: international comparisons reflect flaws and opportunities for better U.S. health care. The Commonwealth Fund website. Available at: https://interactives.commonwealthfund.org/2017/july/mirror-mirror/. Accessed June 3, 2019.

2. Sawyer B, McDermott D. How does the quality of the U.S. healthcare system compare to other countries? Peterson-Kaiser Health System Tracker website. Available at: https://www.healthsystemtracker.org/chart-collection/quality-u-s-healthcare-system-compare-countries/. Accessed June 3, 2019.

3. Institute of Medicine. The future of nursing: leading change, advancing health. Washington, DC: Institute of Medicine; 2010.

4. National Academies of Sciences, Engineering, and Medicine. Assessing progress on the Institute of Medicine Report: the future of nursing. Washington, DC: The National Academies Press; 2016.

5. National Academies of Sciences, Engineering, and Medicine. Project information: the future of nursing 2020-2030. National Academy of Sciences website. Available at: https://www8.nationalacademies.org/pa/projectview.aspx?key=51496. Accessed June 3, 2019.

6. Population Health Agency of Canada. What is the population health approach? Government of Canada website. Available at: https://www.canada.ca/en/public-health/services/health-promotion/population-health/population-health-approach.html. Accessed June 3, 2019.

7. Kindig DA. Understanding population health terminology. Milbank Q 2007;85(1): 139–61. Available at: https://onlinelibrary.wiley.com/doi/abs/10.1111/j.1468-0009. 2007.00479.x.

8. Kindig D, Stoddart G. What is population health? Am J Public Health 2003;93(3): 380–3.

9. American Public Health Association. Health equity. American Public Health Association website. Available at: https://www.apha.org/topics-and-issues/health-equity. Accessed June 3, 2019.

10. Whitehead M. The concepts and principles of equity and health. Health Promot 1991;6(3):217–28.

11. University of Wisconsin Population Health Initiative. County health rankings key findings report. County Health Rankings website. 2018. Available at: http:// www.countyhealthrankings.org/reports/2018-county-health-rankings-key-findings-report. Accessed June 3, 2019.

12. Stevens AB, Aly R. Health policy brief: what is "population health"? Health Policy Institute of Ohio website. Available at: http://www.healthpolicyohio.org/wp-content/uploads/2014/11/WhatIsPopHealth_PolicyBrief.pdf. Accessed June 3, 2019.

13. Merriam-Webster dictionary [Internet]. Advocacy. Available at: https://www. merriam-webster.com/dictionary/advocate. Accessed June 3, 2019.

14. Fowler MD. Social advocacy. Heart Lung 1989;18(1):97–9.

15. Gebbie KM, Wakefield M, Kerfoot K. Nursing and health policy. J Nurs Scholarsh 2000;32(3):307–15.

16. Chaffee MW, Mason DJ, Leavitt JK. A framework for action in policy & politics. In: Mason DJ, Leavitt JK, Chaffee MW, editors. Policy & politics in nursing & health care. St Louis (MO): Elsevier; 2014. p. 1–11.

17. Robert Wood Johnson Foundation. Building a culture of health. Robert Wood Johnson Foundation website. Available at: https://www.rwjf.org/en/cultureofhealth.html/ en/en/taking-action/strengthening-services-and-systems/consumer-experiences. html. Accessed June 3, 2019.

18. American Nurses Association. Ethics and human rights statements. American Nurses Association website. Available at: https://www.nursingworld.org/ ~4af078/globalassets/docs/ana/ethics/ethics-and-human-rights-protecting-and-promoting-final-formatted-20161130.pdf. Accessed June 3, 2019.

19. American Nurses Association. Code of ethics. American Nurses Association website. Available at: https://www.nursingworld.org/coe-view-only. Accessed June 3, 2019.

20. Ballou KA. A historical-philosophical analysis of the professional nurse obligation to participate in sociopolitical activities. Policy Polit Nurs Pract 2000;1(3): 172–84.

21. Fawcett J, Russell G. A conceptual model of nursing and health policy. Policy Polit Nurs Pract 2001;2(2):108–16.

22. Daley K. ANA president Karen Daley tells her needlestick injury story–safe needles save lives [video]. YouTube. Available at: https://www.youtube.com/watch? v=UATLtR_27YE. Accessed June 3, 2019.

23. Milstead JA. Advance practice nurses & public policy, naturally. In: Milstead JA, editor. Health policy and politics: a nurses' guide. Burlington (MA): Jones & Bartlett; 2013. p. 1–27.

24. Longest BE. Health policymaking in the United States. 6th edition. Chicago: Health Administration Press; 2016.

25. Oxford Living Dictionary [Internet]. Media. Available at: https://en.oxforddictionaries.com/definition/media. Accessed June 3, 2019.

26. BusinessDictionary. [Internet]. Media. Available at: http://www.businessdictionary.com/definition/media.html. Accessed June 3, 2019.

27. Mason DJ, Nixon L, Glickstein B, et al. The Woodhull study revisited: nurses' representation in health news media 20 years later. J Nurs Scholarsh 2018;50(6):695–704.

28. Mason DJ, Glickstein B, Westphaln K. Journalists' experiences with using nurses as sources in health news stories. Am J Nurs 2018;118(10):42–50.

Leading Change in Nurse Bedside Shift Report

Ashley Clark, DNP, RN[a],*, Kelly A. Wolgast, DNP, RN[a], Nicole Mazur, MSN, RN[b], Ashley Mekis, MSN, RN, OCN, NE-BC[b]

KEYWORDS

- Bedside shift report • Bedside reporting • Nurse education • Quality improvement
- Patient-centered care

KEY POINTS

- An educational tool kit resource was used to teach registered nurses about bedside report and included a power point, video, practice scenario, and nurse champion education.
- Staff nurses assumed champion roles and are nurses with additional training and were able to be a resource for their coworkers during the implementation phases.
- Bedside nurse shift report was presented in 2 phases to help adaptability and sustainability and included an innovative incentive system.
- Measures were established to gage patient responses to bedside report. A pre- and post-staff survey measured the knowledge and comfort level of the nurses and results used to inform educational needs.
- Leadership buy-in was essential in order to establish nurse bedside shift report as a priority for resourcing and sustainment.

INTRODUCTION

Nurse bedside shift report (NBSR) helps to ensure the safe handoff of care between registered nurses (RNs) by using a structured approach for giving and receiving report and involving the patient and/or support system at the patient's bedside.[1] Evidence shows that NBSR is superior to other methods of nurse-to-nurse shift report and that it has the potential to improve patient safety (falls and medication errors) and the potential to improve patient experiences of care.[1] Even with the evidence, health care facilities can be challenged with successfully implementing and sustaining this change in practice delivery. The purpose is to share a success story on the development, implementation, and sustainment of an NBSR program at a 260-bed acute

[a] College of Nursing, The Pennsylvania State University, 201 Nursing Sciences Building, University Park, PA 16802, USA; [b] Mount Nittany Medical Center, 1800 East Park Avenue, State College, PA 16803, USA
* Corresponding author. College of Nursing, The Pennsylvania State University, 201 Nursing Sciences Building, University Park, PA 16802.
E-mail address: alc316@psu.edu

Nurs Clin N Am 55 (2020) 21–28
https://doi.org/10.1016/j.cnur.2019.10.002
0029-6465/20/© 2019 Elsevier Inc. All rights reserved.

nursing.theclinics.com

care facility. Previous attempts to establish NBSR at this facility, over the past several years, were unsuccessful due to various barriers to change. The program tools and processes are shared with the intent that the lessons learned from this program implementation can be adapted and adopted at other facilities. This project was a successful example of the influence that staff nurses can and do have in implementing care improvement initiatives at the bedside to promote high-quality and safe patient care.

METHODS

Despite previous NBSR attempts in a 260-bed acute care facility, NBSR was not sustained on many patient care units. The inability to sustain NBSR led to an evaluation of the processes used for NBSR education and implementation. The evaluation determined that the processes were not consistent on many patient care units, and buy-in was not achieved on various levels within this facility. The inconsistency led to the formation of an NBSR team, which initially included a unit director, 2 unit supervisors, and a doctoral student who all displayed a strong interest with NBSR. The NBSR team took the lead on gaining buy-in, developing an NBSR educational toolkit and redesigning the NBSR implementation process.

Gaining buy-in is critical to accept and sustain a change in practice delivery. Both formal and informal leaders are needed to support change at all levels within a health care facility, including executive leadership, directors, supervisors, and frontline nursing staff.[2] An NBSR presentation and NBSR-projected timeline were developed and presented to the nursing leadership of this acute care facility to gain initial leadership buy-in.

Educational Resources

Following leadership buy-in, a multimedia educational toolkit, adapted from the Agency for Healthcare Research and Quality (AHRQ), was developed with the purpose to educate, observe, and implement NBSR best practices noted from the NBSR literature.[1] The multimedia educational toolkit for RNs includes NBSR educational PowerPoint, Situation-Background-Assessment-Recommendation-Thank you (SBART) handout, NBSR implementation video, NBSR patient education brochure, and an NBSR role-playing scenario.[3] The NBSR educational PowerPoint included the importance of NBSR, anticipated barriers to NBSR and ways to overcome the barriers, and implementation resources and plans for NBSR. Previous NBSR implementation attempts did not include evidence to support why NBSR is superior to other methods of shift-to-shift report. The SBART handout was given as a resource to standardize and improve communication during NBSR and included specific components that should be included within RN shift report (**Table 1**). The NBSR video displayed nurses implementing the bedside report process, and the role-playing scenario designed for nursing staff provided a shift report that was used for practicing NBSR.

Unit Champions

Following the development of the NBSR educational toolkit, medical-oncology staff RNs were provided with a letter about NBSR to assist with voluntary recruitment of NBSR medical-oncology unit champions. Staff champions are identified in the NBSR literature to serve as role models, trainers, and key change agents during the development and implementation of NBSR.[2,4–8] Six unit champions, representing each of the 3 shifts (7a–3p, 3p–11p, and 11p–7a) were voluntarily recruited. Medical-oncology NBSR unit champions were provided resource binders that included the multimedia educational toolkit. A 4-hour education session led by the

Table 1 SBART tool	
S Situation	"I will be leaving soon, but XXX will be your oncoming nurse that will take great care of you....." Patient name, age, diagnosis, code status, admission status, Name of providers
B Background	"I will be giving report to XXX. Please let us know if you have any questions/concerns." Brief, but pertinent past medical history and any conditions that are having an effect on patient at this time Allergies Admitted for..... Pertinent laboratories/tests Current therapies (treatments, dressings, drains, tubes, IVs, etc.) VS, pain (rating, medications, follow-up) Special needs (alarms, precautions, fall risk, restrictions, etc.) Consults Teaching needs, ask the patient as well..... Discharge plans, ask the patient as well....
A Assessment	Be specific and rReview pertinent ROS Assess all tubes, drains, IVs, dressings, etc. Double check/cosign high-risk medications Scan the environment for safety issues Pertinent tasks completed Any upcoming procedures/tests, etc.
R Recommendation	Review ordered nursing/medical plans of care Any issues going on that need to be resolved Review with patient, patient goals......
T Thanks	Thanks to the patient Answer any questions that patient/family/caregiver/friend may have Does the patient understand the plan of care?

Standard report to streamline the report process used between all nurses at shift change.
Abbreviations: IV, intravenous; ROS, review of systems; VS, vital signs.

NBSR team that used the multimedia education strategies was conducted with the unit champions. Unit champion expectations were discussed for NBSR implementation that included mentoring, supporting, and being a resource for staff RNs (**Box 1**).

RESULTS

An anonymous volunteer RN survey developed by the project team and the education department was sent via an electronic link to staff RNs to gain feedback relating to the acceptability of NBSR. The survey was adapted from concepts drawn from the NBSR literature and included Likert scale and open-ended questions relating to shift report assessment (before NBSR), confidence with NBSR, challenges/ideas to overcome challenges, and nurse demographics.[1] Smartsheet was used to upload and track the anonymous survey responses.[9] The project team and education department had access to the anonymous survey responses. A total of 45 responses out of approximately 70 RNs were collected before NBSR implementation.

Most of the nurses who responded to the survey were bachelors prepared and had been in nursing 6 plus years. Survey results included most of the RNs feeling moderately confident to perform NBSR. One nurse commented, "It's a great idea if it is done

---

Box 1
Champion recruitment letter

Dear _____,

Working together and communicating effectively with patients and families can help improve the quality and safety of hospital care. Communication during transitions in care, such as shift change, is extremely important for ensuring that handoffs are safe and effective. Bedside shift report is a strategy to ensure the safe handoff of care between nurses by involving the patient and/or family at the bedside. Giving patients and families the opportunity to be involved in their plan of care allows them to be a valued partner in the care process.

Bedside shift report can help to improve patient safety and quality, patient experiences of care, nursing staff satisfaction, and time management/accountability between nurses.

As this health care facility advances forward, Nurse Bedside Shift Report is an upcoming initiative to improve the safe handoff for patients. This initiative will take hard work and dedication for implementation and ongoing success. With your knowledge and expertise for improving patient and health care outcomes within this organization, we would like to provide you with the opportunity to become a "Nurse Bedside Shift Report Champion" on the Medical Unit. We would sincerely appreciate the opportunity, if interested, to discuss plans for becoming a champion for this initiative. If interested please contact us by June 5, 2017.

This letter was sent out to registered nurses asking them if they would like to be a champion for their unit and help with the education of the new report process.

correctly and support systems are available to help the patients during shift exchange." Another nurse was apprehensive due to prior unsuccessful attempts stating, "I am hopeful that this will stick on our unit, however I do have doubts due to people not following through after previous initiatives."

On completion of the survey, projected barriers were identified and included time to complete NBSR, health insurance portability and accountability act, attending to patient needs while completing NBSR, and being able to perform NBSR. The survey results, specifically, the concerns about NBSR, emphasized the importance of buy-in from front-line staff. The survey further demonstrated the need for a comprehensive educational platform and continued follow-up to maintain sustainability (**Box 2**).

Implementation Process

The NBSR team and NBSR medical-oncology unit champions assisted with 1-hour NBSR education sessions to medical-oncology staff RNs. These educational sessions were conducted within an education simulation classroom and also on the medical-oncology unit using the educational strategies included within the toolkit.

The redesign of the NBSR implementation process was recommended by leadership to ease the transition into the NBSR process and included piloting NBSR on the medical-oncology care unit in 2 phases. The first phase included introductions, addressing questions and concerns, and scanning the environment for safety issues. The second phase added the use of SBART and the use of the medical record in the patient's room by nursing staff to check laboratory and diagnostic studies, incomplete nursing interventions, and provider orders that still needed to be addressed. The phase approach guided the transition for NBSR implementation and allowed for input from the staff and unit champions along the way.

Box 2
Prepilot RN survey

Ratings: 1 Never, 2 Rarely, 3 Sometimes, 4 Usually, 5 Always
1. Nursing report helps prevent patient safety problems
2. Nursing report helps ensure accountability between nurses
3. Nursing report promotes patient involvement in care
4. Nursing report provides me with a clear picture of my patient assignment
5. Nursing report is completed in a reasonable time frame
6. Nursing report promotes teamwork between shifts
7. Nursing report helps to identify patient teaching needs
   How confident are you in doing bedside shift report?
   1. Not at all confident
   2. Moderately confident
   3. Very confident

Open-ended questions:
   What challenges do you foresee implementing nursing report at the bedside?
   Any ideas that would help to overcome these challenges?

Demographics:
   How many years have you worked in nursing?
      0 to 2, 3 to 5, 6 to 10, 11 to 15, 16+
   What shift do you typically work?
      7 to 3, 7a-7p, 3 to 11, 7p-7a, 11 to 7
   What is the highest level of education you have completed?
      Diploma, Associate, Bachelor's, Master's, Doc

This survey was created in Smartsheet to gage the knowledge of the registered nurse staff before education of bedside nurse shift report.

Feedback Loop

Throughout the pilot, NBSR medical-oncology unit champions served as a resource to mentor and support staff RNs with the NBSR process. The NBSR team or unit supervisors performed random audits 3 times per day across all shifts to monitor for NBSR compliance and mentor RNs. Unit champions and project team members elicited informal staff feedback through discussion to identify barriers and facilitators during the pilot. A follow-up champion meeting occurred during the NBSR pilot to discuss barriers and facilitators to implementation. The informal feedback process aided in the overall success of NBSR implementation because staff input was taken into consideration and changes were made accordingly.

Incentive Program

Unit champions developed an incentive program for RNs that included a point reward system for oncoming/offgoing staff RNs who performed NBSR correctly. The point reward system involved unit supervisors placing "points" within a patient's room that were to be found by staff RNs when completing NBSR. In order to receive the points, both RNs had to be present. The point reward system included point values of 1, 3, or 5 points with prize values worth 5, 10, or 15 points. The incentive program added fun competition to the pilot and was well received by the nursing staff. The nurses with the most points at the end of the pilot earned additional recognition by nursing leadership (**Table 2**).

Table 2 Auditing tool[a]					
Date: Shift: Offgoing RN: Oncoming RN:					
Areas of focus	PT #1	PT #2	PT #3	PT #4	PT #5
RNs go into room					
Introduction					
SBART report					
Safety check					
Goal established					
Whiteboard updated					
Minutes spent in room					

[a] Used to ensure daily compliance with bedside nurse shift report. One random audit complete per shift change by a Clinical Supervisor.
Abbreviations: N/A, the task could not be completed; X, the task was complete.

Postimplementation Survey

After the NBSR pilot, a second anonymous RN survey was conducted to gain insight into the NBSR process. The survey included both Likert scale and open-ended questions relating to shift report assessment (with NBSR), confidence with NBSR, challenges and ideas to overcome challenges, benefits seen with implementing NBSR, and nurse demographics.[1] Benefits realized after NBSR implementation were a new component to this survey. Thirty-eight out of approximately seventy RNs responded to the survey. Most of the nurses who responded to the postpilot survey were bachelors prepared and had been in nursing for 6 plus years.

The survey revealed a moderate amount of confidence with performing NBSR, increased safety associated with NBSR, and an opportunity for strengthening communication with patients and patient support systems. One nurse stated "there are a number of benefits such as increased cooperation among RNs, evaluating the patient environment for cleanliness and safety and patient involvement." Another nurse stated "I think it is important to introduce the oncoming nurse. It also gives you a good idea of what to expect of your assignment." Overtime, patient satisfaction, fall rates during change of shift, and patient safety incidents were monitored during the pilot. Notably, 2 patient safety "catches" were reported, which included the identification of a low oxygenation saturation level and the identification of an incorrect bed alarm setting. A 20% increase in medical-oncology patient satisfaction scores was noted, no falls occurred during the change of shift during the pilot, and overtime did not significantly increase. These results were very positive and encouraging signs that NBSR could have significant positive impact over time on patient care.

DISCUSSION

Following the completion of the NBSR pilot, the pilot results were presented to nursing leadership. The success of the NBSR pilot and ongoing leadership support led to gaining buy-in from the other inpatient unit nurses and leadership. These units included medical-surgical care unit (72 beds), women and children's unit (29 beds), and progressive care unit (32 beds)/intensive care unit (12 beds).

Following unit leader buy-in, NBSR unit champions were voluntarily recruited from each unit across shifts for a total of 20 champions (medical-surgical [11], women's and children's [2], and progressive/intensive care [7]). In addition to staff RNs as NBSR unit champions, some unit supervisors were also recruited as NBSR unit champions for their leadership expertise. A 4-hour NBSR educational session was conducted to orient unit champions to expectations regarding mentoring, supporting, and being a resource for staff RNs. Medical-oncology unit champions involved with the initial project start-up assisted with leading the additional session. The staff auditing tool and incentive program used during the pilot was also shared with the unit directors and unit champions.

Hospital-Wide Education

The project leader, project team members, and NBSR unit champions assisted with 1-hour NBSR education sessions to inpatient RNs. These educational sessions were conducted within an education simulation classroom and also directly on the units using the same educational strategies included during the pilot education. The project team members and the communications department developed an NBSR message for the intranet at the facility to promote the importance of NBSR and the start date for the quality improvement project. This form of communication was effective, as it provided awareness to all employees at this facility.

The NBSR process was disseminated to the remaining in-patient care units in the same 2 phases conducted by the original pilot. Unit directors and supervisor champions randomly audited staff daily for compliance and support during the initial roll-out. The project team randomly audited the NBSR process, rounded with unit supervisors, and elicited informal feedback from staff on the in-patient care units. RN staff feedback from the medical-surgical care unit resulted in the development of an NBSR tip sheet and an SBART handoff tool specific to the medical-surgical care unit. These items were developed by the unit's shared governance council that included an NBSR champion representative.

SUMMARY

Staff nurses at all levels in an acute care facility can and do have a major impact in implementing and sustaining care improvement initiatives at the bedside to promote high-quality and safe patient care. Piloting a care improvement initiative such as NBSR on one in-patient care unit and obtaining informal feedback throughout the process aided in gaining valuable information before the implementation to all inpatient care units. Continuing to obtain informal feedback and periodically evaluating the NBSR process are important considerations for sustainability. In addition to feedback and evaluation, education mechanisms such as educational booster sessions and embedding NBSR education into new staff orientation can also assist with the ongoing success and sustainability of NBSR.

DISCLOSURE

There are no commercial or financial conflicts of interest.

REFERENCES

1. Agency for Healthcare Research and Quality. Nurse bedside shift report: Implementation handbook. 2013. Available at: https://www.ahrq.gov/sites/

default/files/wysiwyg/professionals/systems/hospital/engagingfamilies/strategy3/Strat3_Implement_Hndbook_508.pdf. Accessed June 26, 2017.

2. Boshart B, Knowlton M, Whichello R. Reimplementing bedside shift report at a community hospital. Nurs Manage 2016;47(12):52–5.

3. UP Health System Marquette: A Duke Lifepoint Hospital. Bedside shift report. Available at: https://www.youtube.com/watch?v=RHpbuljThoc. Accessed July 19, 2017.

4. Anderson CD, Mangino RR. Nurse shift report: Who says you can't talk in front of the patient? Nurs Adm Q 2006;30(2):112.

5. Jeffs L, Cardoso R, Beswick S, et al. Enablers and barriers to implementing bedside reporting: Insights from nurses. Nurs Leadersh (Tor Ont) 2013;26(3):39.

6. Hagman J, Oman K, Kleiner C, et al. Lessons learned from the implementation of a bedside handoff model. J Nurs Adm 2013;43(6):315–7.

7. Wakefield DS, Ragan R, Brandt J, et al. Making the transition to nursing bedside shift reports. Jt Comm J Qual Patient Saf 2012;38(6):243.

8. Wollenhaup CA, Stevenson EL, Thompson J, et al. Implementation of a modified bedside handoff for a postpartum unit. J Nurs Adm 2017;47(6):320–6.

9. Smartsheet. Shift report assessment. 2018. Available at: https://smartsheet.com. Accessed August 3, 2017.

Clinical Decision Making at the Bedside

Marie Ann Marino, EdD, RN[a],*, Katherine Andrews, MSN, RN, CCRN[b],
Julia Ward, PhD, RN[a]

KEYWORDS

- Clinical decision making • Experience • Intuition • Information sources
- Environment

KEY POINTS

- Effective decision-making skills by nurses at the bedside are an essential driver of safe, quality care in complex and rapidly changing patient care environments.
- The literature identifies experience, intuition, use of information and sources, and environment as influential to clinical decision making by nurses.
- Clinical decision making by nurses can be enhanced through acknowledgment and support of using intuition in addition to other acceptable sources of knowledge and information.
- Experienced nurses use pattern recognition to facilitate timely and appropriate clinical decisions.
- There are many strategies that can be used in the academic and clinical settings to advance clinical decision-making skills of newly graduated and novice nurses.

INTRODUCTION

Beginning in early childhood, we learn a critical life skill to deal with changes occurring in our world. We learn how to make decisions.[1] Various factors and sources of information influence the decisions we make. These include individuals providing advice, personal knowledge of the subject matter, familiarity with the situation, and potential outcomes that may result from our decisions. As we mature, so too does our capacity to make decisions. Our decision making as a process grows in complexity and so too do the resultant consequences, outcomes, and effect on ourselves and others. Depending on the subject, decision making takes on the persona of the subject. For example, in systems and organizations, executives are held accountable for the viability of their company based on their decision-making capabilities.[2] Similarly, politicians are held accountable for political decisions that affect their constituents. In

[a] Jefferson College of Nursing, Thomas Jefferson University, 901 Walnut Street, Suite 804, Philadelphia, PA 19107, USA; [b] Surgical Intensive Care Unit, Thomas Jefferson University Hospital, 111 South 11th Street, Philadelphia, PA 19107, USA
* Corresponding author.
E-mail address: marie.marino@jefferson.edu

Nurs Clin N Am 55 (2020) 29–37
https://doi.org/10.1016/j.cnur.2019.10.003
0029-6465/20/© 2019 Elsevier Inc. All rights reserved.

nursing.theclinics.com

health care, clinical decision making (CDM) is the term used to describe nursing decisions made in clinical settings. The concept of CDM first appeared in the literature in the 1980s and is defined as the application of distinct thinking patterns and analysis of data at hand along with other influences that nurses and other health professionals use to make judgements about the care they provide to patients.[3,4] CDM, particularly by nurses, remains a major area of scientific inquiry today because of its relationship to health care quality and safety. The literature is replete with studies and reviews that relate to how nurses make decisions in the fast-paced, rapidly changing health care environment.[5]

MODELS OF CLINICAL DECISION MAKING

Several models of CDM can be found in the literature. Two of the most commonly applied and investigated are Benner's "from novice to expert" model[3,6] and Tanner's clinical judgment model.[5] Benner's[3,6] model is an intuitive, humanistic decision-making model by which nurses move through 5 stages of skill acquisition as they develop clinical competence: novice, advanced beginner, competent, proficient, and expert. Advancement among the stages depends on skill performance and decision making. Nurses advance from earlier stages where there is reliance on abstract principles to later stages where use of past, concrete principles and recognition of relationships and patterns are hallmarks.

Tanner's clinical judgment model[5] provides a conceptual understanding of CDM and posits that clinical judgements are made through 4 aspects: noticing, interpreting, responding, and reflecting. According to Tanner, judgments are made by experienced nurses through gaining a perceptual grasp of the situation (noticing), developing a sufficient understanding (interpreting), deciding on whether or not to act and how to act (responding), and getting a "read" on how the patient is responding to the intervention (reflecting). This process is followed by a review of the outcomes of the clinical judgment(s) made.

Two additional models that have been widely used to understand the process of CDM are the systematic–positivist model and the intuitive–humanistic model.[7,8] The systematic–positivist model describes CDM as a systematic process reliant on theoretic knowledge to analyze data and form a diagnosis. It asserts that human responses to health and illness can be can be broken down into smaller components and then identified, measured, and understood. The intuitive–humanistic model,[7,8] influenced by Benner's[3,6] work, asserts that intuition is an essential component of clinical judgment and is linked to the nurse's experience. The 6 aspects of this model related to intuitive judgment are: pattern recognition, similarity recognition, common sense understanding, skilled know-how, use of salience, and deliberative rationality.[7,8] The model emphasizes that intuitive judgment relies more on a one's perception of the situation than scientific evidence-based knowledge. These models offer a foundation for understanding how nurses make decisions in the clinical setting and provide a framework for scientific inquiry.

KEY FACTORS ASSOCIATED WITH CLINICAL DECISION MAKING

An exploration of the literature revealed that there are several key factors associated with CDM: experience, intuition, use of information and sources, and environment.

Experience

Experience is a key contributor to CDM. According to Benner,[3] experience is a process of knowing whereby repeated exposures to situations lead to a refinement of earlier thoughts and ideas. These exposures enable nurses to build a collection of cognitive resources upon which they can reflect and use to interpret data. Experience is critical to the development of clinical decision-making competency. The relationship between experience and CDM has been explored in the literature.[9–12]

Stinson[11] examined the relationships among clinical experience and CDM in a descriptive correlational study of registered nurses currently used in a critical care environment. Using a convenience sample (n = 413) drawn from the membership of the American Association of Critical Care Nurses (AACN) (N = 94,000), CDM was measured using the Clinical Decision Making in Nursing Scale (CDMNS).[13] The CDMNS is a 40 question, Likert-type (from 5 [strongly agree] to 1 [strongly disagree]), self-report instrument used to identify and evaluate CDM in nursing. The scale contains 4 subscales: (1) search for alternatives or options, (2) canvassing of objectives and values, (3) evaluation and reevaluation of consequences, and (4) search for information and unbiased assimilation of new information. Instrument scores can range from 40 (negative perception of decision making) to 200 (higher perception of decision making). Cronbach's alpha reliability coefficient for the CDMNS is reported at 0.83. Stinson's[11] sample consisted of registered nurses used in a critical care unit (intensive care unit, cardiac care unit, postanesthesia unit) who were primarily classified as experts in general nursing (83.1%) and critical care (75.1%) experience on Benner's classification system.[3] Data revealed that there were no significant differences seen in CDMNS scores among Benner's[3] experience categories but that the sample, as a whole, had a higher mean score (152.6) than most samples reported in the literature. The findings suggest that using a professional organization to obtain the study sample may have caused an overrepresentation of nurses with advanced levels of experience and that critical care nurses with significant clinical experience have higher CDM skills.

The ability to recognize cues in a patient situation and intervene in a timely manner and appropriately is a hallmark of expert clinical practice and foundational to CDM. Burbach and Thompson[10] conducted an integrative review of literature published between 1964 and 2013 to describe factors influencing cue recognition by undergraduate nursing students in real and simulated clinical environments and evidence of the differences between novice and expert nurses' cue recognition. The authors operationally defined the term *cue* as a piece of objective or subjective information and *cue recognition* as the acknowledgment of the presence of objective or subjective patient data by nurses. Using the search terms of *cue, cue recognition, clinical cue,* and *clinical reasoning*, sources were identified and included whether they sampled undergraduate or newly graduated nurses. The sampling strategy was later expanded to include experienced nurses as well owing to the low number of studies that met the initial criteria. A total of 21 studies were selected for inclusion and included both quantitative (n = 12) and qualitative (n = 9) methodologies. Differences in cue recognition between undergraduate or newly graduated nurses and expert nurses emerged as a general theme from the analysis. Novice nurses were reported to have gathered fewer cues overall compared with expert nurses and demonstrated difficulty differentiating between relevant and irrelevant cues. Also, undergraduate nursing students tended to assign equal weights to cues and consider cues in a sequence, leading to missed cue recognition or discounting relevant cues. Alternatively, expert nurses with higher levels of experience demonstrated greater accuracy and efficiency in cue recognition and clustered cues when forming clinical judgments.

Similarly, Nibbelink and Brewer[9] conducted an integrative review to identify indicators of CDM by registered nurses in medical-surgical environments. Using the terms *decision making, nurses, process, decision making, clinical,* and *nursing practice,* the search strategy yielded a total of 17 articles published between 1998 and 2015 and included both quantitative design (n = 3), qualitative design (n = 9), and systematic review (n = 5) studies. A key theme identified included that clinical judgments made by nurses were more influenced by previous clinical experiences with patients than by the current clinical situation in which decisions are made. Experience enabled nurses to see patterns among patients that increase understanding of patient status and situation awareness. Further, that experience was associated with factors such as confidence, intuition, use of protocols, and collaboration with colleagues.

These findings provide evidence that the experienced nurse is able to solicit knowledge needed to make a clinical decision by drawing on past experiences with like situations and typical response patterns from previous patient encounters. This finding is directly aligned with Tanner's clinical judgment model,[5] which posits that clinical experience increases the cognitive resources necessary for CDM and supports nurses' interpretation of clinical data and the decision of which course of action to take.

Intuition

Evidence-based practice (EBP) is recognized as an essential component in the provision of safe, quality patient care. EBP, through integration of best research evidence, clinical expertise, patient preference, and values, strengthens CDM.[14] CDM is guided by best evidence when clinicians turn to best practice guidelines, clinical pathways, or algorithms. Although it is readily accepted that EBP is associated with delivering high-quality care, nurses often report that they continue to rely on intuition as an integral part of their decision-making process.[15] The nursing decision-making process uses complex critical thinking skills that involve both analytical and intuitive judgments based on patient needs and the current situation.[16] With a significant focus on EBP, the value of intuition as an integral part of the decision-making process has been underrated. Current review of literature, however, validates the use of experienced nursing intuition as an important part of effective decision making. Intuition by nurses has been shown to support high-quality, safe patient care at the bedside.[17]

The Merriam-Webster Dictionary defines intuition as "the power or faculty of attaining to direct knowledge or cognition without evident rational thought and inference. Other common definitions of intuition include a feeling without reasoning, decision making with limited concrete information, or an understanding without logic."[18] Concepts associated with intuition include having a gut feeling, sixth sense, or hunch. Alternately, Pearson[19] posited that intuition can be considered a cognitive skill rather than merely an abstract hunch or feeling because it involves pattern recognition in which expert clinicians draw from similar and previous experiences.

Research indicates that intuition in nursing practice develops over time and is based on the knowledge and experience of caring for patients in the clinical setting. Melin-Johansson and colleagues[18] conducted an integrative review composed of both quantitative (n = 5) and qualitative (n = 11) studies to examine registered nurses' intuition in the clinical setting, nursing process, and relationships. Data from the studies was drawn from 2575 nurses working in acute, critical, and emergent care settings. Results indicated a positive relationship between number of years of experience and sense of intuition. Further, that length of experience was the most significant factor determining a nurse's reliance on intuition in CDM. Other factors related to a nurses' ability to develop and use intuition in the clinical setting included application of the skill and assertiveness and in relationships with patients include having a unique connection with patients, certain psychological and physical responses, and personal characteristics, like openness, vulnerability, and emotional availability. Application of intuition during the nursing process was more commonly applied during the assessment and implementation phases and when making a nursing diagnosis.[18]

Although intuition is viewed as an experience- and knowledge-based approach to decision making associated with enhanced clinical judgment, effective decision making, and crisis aversion, its use is often undervalued among health care providers.[17] This is primarily due to the abstract terms used to describe it and that intuition is based on the knowledge and understanding of the observer rather than scientific evidence.[18] However, intuition skill development and its effective use in nursing practice have been reported in the literature. Nalliah[20] reports there are certain situations in which intuition-based decision making can be highly effective and may actually result in a better final decision than an evidence-based decision. These circumstances include when a clinical situation lacks sufficient evidence, has time constraints requiring a rapid decision, or involves a complex or ambiguous problem. Under these circumstances, expert health care providers who draw from experience and pattern recognition sense a solution before a structured decision-making process ensues.

Use of Information and Sources

EBP is recognized as an essential component in the provision of safe, high-quality patient care. EBP integrates best research evidence, clinical expertise, patient preference, and values into clinical care and strengthens CDM by clinicians.[14] And although significantly better outcomes are associated with EBP, it is still not used by most nurses and other clinicians as standard clinical practice. Additionally, although the mastery of skills necessary to work within an EBP framework is emphasized in most academic nursing programs, the literature demonstrates that integration of best evidence into standard patient care by newly graduated nurses is poor.[21,22] Marshall and colleagues[22] used a case study design to explore critical care nurses' perceptions of the usefulness and accessibility of information sources used to make clinical decisions. Data indicated that nurse participants preferred to seek information from those individuals with greater levels of experience or relevant specific expertise. This preference was particularly strong in situations of clinical uncertainty. Print- and electronic-based information sources were infrequently identified as useful. A problematic finding was that both bedside nurses and senior clinical nurse leaders revealed that basing clinical practice on best evidence was not useful in making clinical decisions.

Although there are a variety of knowledge sources available to nurses for use in CDM, using colleagues as a source of useful information when making clinical decisions is widely described as a preferred resource in the literature.[21,23–25] In an ethnographic study of 9 newly graduated nurses (range, 9–20 months of clinical experience), Voldbjerg and colleagues[21] used participant-observation and semistructured individual interviews to collect data on the use of knowledge sources in CDM. Newly graduated nurses' use of knowledge sources in CDM emerged within 3 main themes: other, oneself, and gut feeling. Nurses with experience ("other") were seen as an imperative knowledge source and were sought first when novice nurses were confronted with a problem or unfamiliar procedure. None of the novice nurses were assigned a specific mentor but described using experienced nurses as unofficial mentors or "sounding boards," particularly when they had previous positive experience soliciting advice from them. Advice was sought from experienced nurses when there was an inconsistency between what newly graduated nurses were told and what they thought to be acceptable in a given patient care situation.

Interchanges between novice and experienced nurses were observed to be informal and limited to an explanation of how to do something, rather than referencing evidence or guidelines and explicating the why something was being done in a particular way. Additional sources of knowledge included physicians, patients, and family. Voldbjerg and colleagues[21] found that, although newly graduated nurses used clinical guidelines, procedures, and standards as a knowledge source, interviews revealed that the decision to do so was task based and influenced by an experienced nurse telling them to do so. Use of oneself as a knowledge source, through patterns and personal and professional experience, was deemed an essential component of practice by newly graduated nurses, but articulation and reflection after the decision/task were challenging. Last, a gut feeling was used in situations of uncertainty and when newly graduated nurses were in situations where it was difficult to determine the right way to proceed.[21]

Environment

The environment in which a nurse works influences overall CDM.[11] There are many contextual elements that make up the culture of a work environment and these can either support or inhibit effective CDM by nurses. According to the AACN,[26] effective decision making is 1 of 6 essential standards that produce effective and sustainable outcomes for nurses and patients. A critical element of effective decision making is that health care organizations clearly articulate the organization's values and that team members incorporate these values into CDM. To evaluate the current status of the nurse work environment and integration of the 6 standards, the AACN launched its most recent study to evaluate the relationship between the nurse and the environment in which they provide patient care.[27] The mixed methods study of 8080 AACN members indicated that the health of the nurse work environment has improved since its previous environment study in 2013.[28] Specifically, that nurses have opportunities to influence decisions that affect the quality of patient care was ranked by nurses as 1 of the 5 highest work unit elements, up from 2013.

Additional contextual factors in the nurse work environment impact the CDM ability of nurses, including relationships with peers and leadership, time constraints, workload, resources, and interruptions.[29–31] A meta-review by Francke and colleagues[29] revealed that a lack of support from peers or supervisors negatively influenced a nurse's decision to implement best practice guidelines. Time constraints and workload are also described as environmental factors influencing CDM. Not having an adequate amount of time is reported to negatively influence a nurse's ability to make sound clinical decisions.[30] Additionally, heavy patient assignments or distribution of workload impact the availability of time and contribute to compromises in CDM, specifically choosing less than optimal decisions or interventions.[31] A unit with inadequate resources (human and material) impacts the work environment and diminishes the time available for high-quality decision making.[30] Interruptions have an adverse impact on CDM by nurses and other health professionals by affecting the cognitive ability to accurately recall information and make effective clinical decisions. Interruptions include being asked questions by others, having others ask for assistance, phone calls, or others wanting to exchange information.[31]

IMPLICATIONS FOR NURSE LEADERS AND EDUCATORS

The development of competence in skills needed to make effective and high-quality decisions is an area of major inquiry in the literature. Given that the literature clearly supports that newly graduated nurses perceive their academic preparation as insufficient for making clinical decisions in their current role, continued development of CDM skills is critical. Several strategies can be used both in the academic setting and in clinical practice to facilitate and advance CDM skills of nurses at the bedside.

The use of intuition in clinical practice as an acceptable part of the decision-making process should be an area of focus for nurse educators and nurse leaders. All decisions cannot be made based on current best evidence; therefore, it is critical that nurse educators understand the concept of intuition and its role in CDM. It is essential that students learn in environments that support the development and refinement of intuition as an adjunct to CDM. More clinical experiences and simulations are needed to enhance this skill in undergraduate students. Expanding the use of simulation scenarios that challenge student's clinical judgment and reasoning and the use of intuition should be incorporated throughout the academic program. Debriefing and reflection should be used to facilitate students' development of insight into their own critical thinking. Feedback and coaching should direct students to recognize decision making that leads to a "failure to notice" and factors in the situation that may have contributed to that failure.

Given the correlation between length of nursing experience and increased sense and use of intuition, further support and development of intuitive skills are central to the progression of the newly graduated and novice nurses. Health care organizations should acknowledge and support intuition, in addition to use of other acceptable sources of knowledge and information, as an important part of nurses' clinical practice. Use of experienced nurses by novice nurses as a reputable and acceptable source of knowledge, often before or as an alternative to best evidence, indicates an area of opportunity in the clinical environment. In the academic setting, educators should increase focus on skills and competencies needed to work within an evidence-based framework, including critical reflection of simulated and in vivo patient encounters, formulation of problems, searching, retrieving, and evaluating research evidence. In the clinical setting, assignment of official mentors to newly graduated and novice nurses, particularly ones that can communicate information based on best evidence, can serve to reinforce use of appropriate knowledge sources and demonstrate integration of evidence and clinical guidelines into safe, quality patient care. Facilitating experienced nurse's reinforcement of EBP principles when mentoring and/or precepting new and novice nurses can be instrumental in their adoption of EBP as a framework for practice. Additionally, the literature clearly demonstrates a correlation between the environment within which nurses work and CDM. Nursing leaders can create a work environment culture that supports high-quality CDM by advocating for adequate resources; promoting positive, healthy interpersonal relationships among staff; fostering open and honest communication; and supporting the development of CDM skills.

SUMMARY

The complexity and rapidly changing environment of health care place significant pressure on nurses in clinical settings. How nurses make decisions within this environment have significant implications to patient care outcomes. CDM has been an area of significant inquiry in the literature and several key factors emerge as influencers of CDM at the bedside, including experience, intuition, use of information and sources, and environment. Further work is needed to explore how these and others factors affect the quality of decisions made by nurses and the impact of those decisions on patient care. Additional work is needed to understand how these factors will interface with technologically supported decision aids and applications. Last, several strategies can be used by nurse educators and leaders to facilitate newly graduated and novice nurses' development of effective CDM skills and establish environments that support ideal decision making by nurses.

REFERENCES

1. Demirtaş VY, Sucuoğlu H. In the early childhood period children's decision-making processes. Procedia Social and Behavioral Sciences 2009;1(1):2317–26.
2. Buchanan L, O'Connell A. A brief history of decision making. Harv Bus Rev 2006; 84(1):32–41.
3. Benner PE. From novice to expert: excellence and power in clinical nursing practice. Menlo Park (CA): Addison-Wesley Pub. Co., Nursing Division; 2001.
4. Bakalis N, Watson R. Nurses' decision-making in clinical practice. Nurs Stand 2005;19(23):33–9.
5. Tanner C. Thinking like a nurse: a research-based model of clinical judgment in nursing. J Nurs Educ 2006;45:204–11.
6. Benner PE. Using the Dreyfus model of skill acquisition to describe and interpret skill acquisition and clinical judgment in nursing practice and education. Bull Sci Technol Soc 2004;24(3):188–99.
7. Krishnan P. A philosophical analysis of clinical decision making in nursing. J Nurs Educ 2018;57(2):73–8.
8. Banning M. A review of clinical decision making: models and current research. J Clin Nurs 2008;17(2):187–95.
9. Nibbelink CW, Brewer BB. Decision-making in nursing practice: an integrative literature review. J Clin Nurs 2018;27(5–6):917–28.
10. Burbach BE, Thompson SA. Cue recognition by undergraduate nursing students: an integrative review. J Nurs Educ 2014;53(9 Suppl):S73–81.
11. Stinson KJ. Benner's framework and clinical decision-making in the critical care environment. Nurs Sci Q 2017;30(1):52–7.
12. Johansen ML, O'Brien JL. Decision making in nursing practice: a concept analysis. Nurs Forum 2016;51(1):40–8.
13. Jenkins HM. A research tool for measuring perceptions of clinical decision making. J Prof Nurs 1985;1(4):221–9.
14. Melnyk BM, Gallagher-Ford L, Long LE, et al. The establishment of evidence-based practice competencies for practicing registered nurses and advanced practice nurses in real-world clinical settings: proficiencies to improve healthcare quality, reliability, patient outcomes, and costs. Worldviews Evid Based Nurs 2014;11(1):5–15.
15. Chilcote DR. Intuition: a concept analysis. Nurs Forum 2017;52(1):62–7.
16. Miller EM, Hill PD. Intuition in clinical decision making: differences among practicing nurses. J Holist Nurs 2018;36(4):318–29.
17. Robert RR, Tilley DS, Petersen S. A power in clinical nursing practice: concept analysis on nursing intuition. Medsurg Nurs 2014;23(5):343–9.
18. Melin-Johansson C, Palmqvist R, Ronnberg L. Clinical intuition in the nursing process and decision-making-A mixed-studies review. J Clin Nurs 2017;26(23–24): 3936–49.
19. Pearson H. Science and intuition: do both have a place in clinical decision making? Br J Nurs 2013;22:212–5.
20. Nalliah RP. Clinical decision making - choosing between intuition, experience and scientific evidence. Br Dent J 2016;221(12):752–4.

21. Voldbjerg SL, Gronkjaer M, Wiechula R, et al. Newly graduated nurses' use of knowledge sources in clinical decision-making: an ethnographic study. J Clin Nurs 2017;26(9–10):1313–27.
22. Marshall AP, West SH, Aitken LM. Preferred information sources for clinical decision making: critical care nurses' perceptions of information accessibility and usefulness. Worldviews Evid Based Nurs 2011;8(4):224–35.
23. Spenceley S, O'Leary K, Chizawsky-Fee L, et al. Sources of information used by nurses to inform practice: an integrative review. Int J Nurs Stud 2008;45(6): 954–70.
24. Marshall AP, West SH, Aitken LM. Clinical credibility and trustworthiness are key characteristics used to identify colleagues from whom to seek information. J Clin Nurs 2013;22(9–10):1424–33.
25. O'leary DF, Mhaolrúnaigh SN. Information seeking behaviour of nurses: where is information sought and what processes are followed? J Adv Nurs 2012;68(2): 379–90.
26. Nurses AAoC-C. AACN standards for establishing and sustaining healthy work environments: a journey to excellence. 2nd edition. Aliso Viejo (CA): American Association of Critical-Care Nurses; 2016.
27. Ulrich B, Barden C, Cassidy L, et al. Critical care nurse work environments 2018: findings and implications. Crit Care Nurse 2019;39(2):67–84.
28. Ulrich BT, Lavandero R, Woods D, et al. Critical care nurse work environments 2013: a status report. Crit Care Nurse 2014;34(4):54–79.
29. Francke A, Smit MC, de Veer AJ, et al. Factors influencing the implementation of clinical guidelines for health care professionals: a systematic meta-review. BMC Med Inform Decis Mak 2008;8(1):38.
30. Ten Ham W, Ricks EJ, Van Rooyan D, et al. An integrative literature review of the factors that contribute to professional nurses and midwives making sound clinical decisions. Int J Nurs Knowl 2015;28(1):19–29.
31. Smith M, Higgs J, Ellis E. Factors influencing clinical decision making. In: Higgs J, Jones M, Loftus S, et al, editors. Clinical reasoning in the health professions. 3rd edition. Sydney (Australia): Butterworth-Heinemann; 2008. p. 89–100.

Making Good Use of Your Limited Time
Supporting Novice Nurses

Sheri Matter, PhD, RN, MSN, MBA, MS, NEA-BC*,
Kelly A. Wolgast, DNP, RN

KEYWORDS

- Novice nurse • Efficiency • Tools • Precepting • Time management • Benner
- Stacking • Technology

KEY POINTS

- Developing a tool kit to provide safe and efficient care is pivotal for the novice nurse's successful transition to a competent nurse.
- Embracing personal support elevates the novice nurse's level of efficiency and provides opportunity to build a tool kit for the future. Personal support may include relationships with peers, such as mentors, and teamwork as well as length and type of orientation.
- System supports include efficiency mechanisms, such as electronic medical records, smart pumps, and a systems approach of providing care.

INTRODUCTION

Novice nurses join the professional work force from a variety of schools, programs, and experiences. Based on Patricia Benner's[1] novice to expert framework, the phases of nursing competence are developed through experience. The levels of competency include novice, advanced beginner, competent, proficient, and expert.[1] Achieving the highest level of competency in practice, an expert nurse is one who has a full understanding of the entire situation surrounding patient care.[1] As new nurse's successful progression from novice to advanced beginner to becoming clinically competent is achieved with proper planning and development of personal and systems support.

Nursing efficiency is vitally connected to the solvency, or financial health, of any health care organization. Economic factors play an influencing role in today's hospital staffing. Health care has reached a new era of cost containment that is combined with the expectation of quality outcomes. As the strain of economic pressure increases in health care organizations, the accountability for meeting the measures of triple aim

College of Nursing, The Pennsylvania State University, Nursing Sciences Building, University Park, PA 16802, USA
* Corresponding author.
E-mail address: sxm1898@psu.edu

Nurs Clin N Am 55 (2020) 39–49
https://doi.org/10.1016/j.cnur.2019.10.004
0029-6465/20/© 2019 Elsevier Inc. All rights reserved.

increases.[2] This accountability creates a greater sense of urgency for efficient high-quality patient care. Triple aim is the accountability program that can affect a health care organization's level of reimbursement by Medicare and insurers.[2] According to the Institute for Healthcare Improvement, organizations that achieve triple aim have a healthier population when patients have less complex care, high-quality care, and satisfied patient experience at a lower per-patient cost.[3] Ensuring that quality measures are met in a cost-effective manner is included in the role of every bedside nurse and nursing leader.

Delivering high-quality care to meet patient expectations in a cost-effective manner is a skill that nurses need to learn early in their career. Nurses often are the largest line item in the salary budgets of health care systems, and hospitals function on the policy of producing the highest quality care at optimal cost.[4] Novice nurses who combine learning efficiency with high-quality compassionate care create success for their careers and play a vital role in the success of their organization.

During the orientation period, it is important for novice nurses to gather tools to apply throughout their career. A tool kit can help establish a foundation built during the novice stage and further develop through advanced beginner to competence. The tools that support nurses are as diverse as their portals of entry into the nursing field and range from support systems to technology. Each day in a nurse's life is varied by patient care requirements; therefore, the tools need to be as diverse as the situations encountered when entering practice. Huntington and colleagues[5] in a quantitative study assessing nurses' work-life balance noted that little has changed to support nurses' time management both personally and organizationally while health care has become more complex. In 2003, Waterworth[6] adeptly addressed the issue of time management and efficiency strategies. Little information was noted at that time and little research or evidence has been added to the literature since Waterworth's work addressing time management skills.[6]

The role of the nursing leader is instrumental when guiding the transition of novice nurses to advanced beginner nurses. Strategies and lessons learned in this article are shared through the experiences of 2 seasoned nursing executives with more than 60 years of combined leadership experience. Leaders play a pivotal role in supporting the personal and systems support for novice nurses' success. Nursing leaders set the tone for preceptors and mentors as well as ensure that the systems are supporting the team as intended.

DISCUSSION

This article presents elements of both personal and systems support for creating an efficient competent nurse from a novice nurse. The initial focus is on onboarding and self-help. Personal or individual support includes areas, such as precepting, nurse residency programs, mentorship, and self-management. The latter part of the article addresses systems support elements, such as technology and organizational structure, including the role of information technology through decision support and protocols. The Kellogg logic model serves as a visual representation of the development pathway of the novice nurse to supporting the mission and the outcomes of the organization.[7]

ORIENTATION—ONBOARDING
Precepting

A novice nurse's orientation with a preceptor is part of the foundation for efficiency and competency for a new career and within the current system of employment. A

40-year-old concept, precepting has become the cornerstone of the onboarding process for most novice nurses.[4] Adequately trained preceptors are critical for novice nurses' transition from student to advanced beginner nurse. Novice nurses are noted as graduating from the entry-level education but lacking prioritization and time management skills.[1] Precepting affords new nurses time to learn routines, develop critical thinking, and develop time management skills by learning from the efficiency of their preceptors.[8] A supportive environment is critical when developing the efficiency of the novice nurse. As leaders choose and assign preceptors, it is important that the preceptors are contemporary, embrace personal and systems supports for gaining efficiency, and know how to pass along those strategies and skills to novice nurses.

Nurse Residency or Extended Orientation Programs

Nurse residency programs or extended transition programs have been shown to improve nurses' transiting into advanced beginner nurses. Programs can range from 6 months to 6 years and are noted to improve planning, prioritizing, communication, and leadership, creating an efficient advanced beginner nurse.[9] Through the early development of efficiency skills, time management is an unintended benefit of a formalized and lengthened onboarding program. Nurse residency programs have varied formats and there is little to no evidence as to which type of program is best. What is known is that a longer orientation program creates greater success for novice nurses.[9] Baumann and colleagues,[9] in a cross-sectional study comparing nurses who participated in an extended transition program to nurses who did not participate, found that an extended orientation benefited novice nurses in practice and reduced turnover.[9] With that success comes efficiency and improves key dimensions of care.

Mentorship

There are health care organizations that have formal mentoring programs whereas others have no mentoring programs. Mentors have been shown to improve becoming part of the culture on nursing units.[10] Mentors who are self-selected fit the needs of the new nurse. Mentors can support a novice nurse's emotional needs as well as provide tips on how to best provide care. The use of a mentor often is part of a nurse's transition after the initial orientation program. When asked, many nurses articulate that formal or informal mentors helped transition them to be successful efficient nurses.[10] Mentors are known to develop a nurse's ability to think critically and support efficiency.[10] This leads to the nurse becoming part of the high functioning team, and nurses who work with others find efficiency making overwhelming situations manageable.[10]

Stacking

Kohtz[11] addressed the concept of stacking as the "dynamic and complex cognitive process which involves decision making, organizing, and reorganizing based on the patient's needs." Improving these skills decreases stress, especially in new nurses, and contributes to a healthy work environment on the nursing unit.[11] Multiple studies found that during transition, time management was among the most distressing concerns.[11] Preceptors and nursing leaders play a role in helping novice nurses learn the skill of coordination of care supporting quality of care and efficiency.[11] The manager plays a large role by influencing factors, such as unit schedules, interruptions, and developing delegation.[11] Preceptors play an important role in teaching delegation and point-of-care (POC) documentation.[11] Shaw and colleagues,[8] in a mixed methods study, found supporting evidence that enhanced learning opportunities in prioritization and time management serve newly graduated nurses and their future patients well and support the need for leaders and preceptors to develop stacking skills.

Self-Management

Among nurses working in hospitals in the United States, 11% are prone to long hours.[9] According to Stone and Treloar,[12] long hours contribute to stress, high blood pressure, unhealthy diets, depression, work injuries, diabetes, and cardiovascular disease. Kirkwood[13] found that decreased sleep and long, frequent shifts without rest lead to harmful health effects. Long and frequent shifts should be avoided to preserve all nurses' health and protect patient outcomes. Significant breaks, including meal breaks, are instrumental during a nurse's shift to boost health and promote mindfulness.[14] Mindfulness is the quality of attention and can be achieved when the mind is not allowed to wander.[14] This can be achieved only when employees take breaks from the work and allow themselves time to refocus.[14] Caring for self goes a long way when caring for others. Tired, stressed nurses are not as efficient in providing quality patient care.

Time Management

Time management skills are developed throughout a nurse's career. The foundation of time management can be developed through preceptors, mentors, teamwork, and time spent delivering nursing care. The unpredictability of nursing activities challenges time management and the creation of efficiency. The tools of quality improvement can support the role of time management. There is a need to establish a routine, set priorities, coordinate care (including the team), and avoid interruptions.[6,15] Routines can be supported through shared decision making at the unit level in scheduled care routines and multidisciplinary patient rounds. Examples of routines include tasks, such as reviewing laboratory data, medication administration, rounding, and hand-offs of patient care.[16] Finding a routine can help establish a pattern to a nurse's day and create a sense of familiarity.

Nurses have identified confidence in time management and prioritization, including delegation skills that can be developed through exposure.[16] Exposure to difficult situations and how to navigate through them in a timely manner can be grounded in the novice nurse's orientation. The support of preceptors, nurse residency programs, and mentors is valuable when developing time management skills. Bergman and Shubert[16] found that there is increased confidence with frequent exposure supported by simulation and supportive periods, such as orientation.

SYSTEMS

Just as there are individual supports in developing efficiencies for a nurse, there are systems approaches. These approaches include processes, teamwork, and technology. **Fig. 1** is a schematic of the tools that the novice nurse may build on to become an advanced beginner nurse. A logic model is a visual that presents how resources support the plan and change results to achieve sought-after outcomes. This model includes resources/inputs, activities, outputs, outcomes, and impact. The input is the nurse's education, which varies from nurse to nurse. The activities include systematic inputs as well as inputs that are personal to the nurse. Outputs include efficient and competent care. The outcomes are measured by patient outcomes as well as nurses who find satisfaction in their work. Outcomes lead to the impact of an organization that supports the mission with the competent efficient nurse.[7]

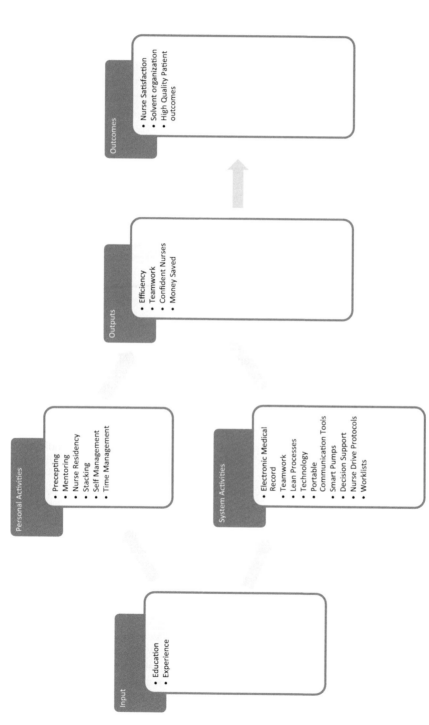

Fig. 1. Logic model. (*Data from* Using logic models to bring together planning, evaluation, and action: Logic model development guide. W. K. Kellogg Foundation. https://www.wkkf.org/resource-directory/resource/2006/02/wk-kellogg-foundation-logic-model-development-guide Published February 2, 2006. Accessed on April 1, 2019.)

The outcomes are the focus of the systems support for novice nurses. When a nurse reaches competence and can efficiently and independently navigate the day, the nurse has more satisfaction from work.[1] A nurse's experiences and tools needed from a tool kit for care activities are different daily because each day presents with different patients and diagnoses. Understanding the process within the logic model allows the nurse to envision what is needed to efficiently work through their days during the beginning of a career. This growth can provide the new nurse satisfaction and confidence to move toward competency.

Teamwork

Teamwork is instrumental to creating efficiency in health care systems. Chan and colleagues[17] found that registered nurses support each other when there are heavy workloads and they are quick to rescue. Teamwork is a part of the unit culture and not a learned response of the nurse. Included in teamwork is delegation, which is a difficult skill to learn as a novice nurse. It often is difficult to delegate care when a nurse is not yet personally comfortable with the care the nurse is delivering. Delegation is something that needs to be worked on during the orientation period and beyond. This can be difficult because novice nurses are developing their own competencies.[9] The future of nursing report by the Institute of Medicine states that nurses must work at the top of their license.[18] This improves the novice nurse's ability to perform the registered nurse–only tasks in a safe and timely manner.[18] Through learned delegation techniques, novice nurses working at the top of their license contribute to the team at the highest level.

Multidisciplinary Rounds

Multidisciplinary rounds are a systems approach to efficiency. Although often seen as an interruption, multidisciplinary rounds can create efficiency if well planned.[19] Planned rounds decrease interruptions and allow nurses to prioritize and plan their day.[19] An added efficiency is to welcome a patient's family to be present during rounds to help increase timely communication with the family and advance continuity of care. Physicians report fewer interruptions by nurses, families, and supportive departments, such as pharmacy and physical therapy, when engaging in multidisciplinary rounds.[19] By having rounds at scheduled times, all parties involved can better plan the activities for the day. All members of the health care team discuss the plan of care and have a clear consistent plan for the patient. Routine rounding also supports a planned discharge that creates efficiency for nurses and patients and sets expectations to support the patient experience and outcomes.[20] Rounds must be well planned, follow a structured process, and stay within a time limit to create a focused meaningful process. Cornell and colleagues,[19] through a time motion study, found that nurses and physicians who invest in the process see value and develop an understanding of questions to expect and what is to be addressed at the time of the rounding.

Processes—Lean Management Systems

There are quality-improvement processes that focus on efficiencies and decrease waste. One example is the Lean principles based on the Toyota system.[21] Virginia Mason Medical Center is an example of a health care organization that applies the Toyota principles to transform care delivery.[21] Recognizing the changing health care reimbursement system, the organization embraced the Lean way of thinking to provide efficient high-quality patient care. Based on the concepts that there are 7 types of waste, including time, motion, inventory, processing, defects, transportation, and overproduction, processes throughout the organization have been reworked to avoid waste.[21] Lean organizations create efficiencies by implementing supportive systems and avoiding overproduction. This is valuable to the novice nurse because Lean processes have fewer steps and consistently promote the delivery of high-quality care in the same simplistic way. Virginia Mason experienced fiscally responsible staffing with high-quality outcomes and high patient experience scores after beginning in the process in 2001 and achieved positive results within 4 years of process deployment.[21] Positive results encourage staff involvement in identifying and presenting areas of waste as part of their employment expectations.[21]

Lean principles are being adopted by a growing number of health care organizations.[22] Due to the growing financial pressures of health care systems, health care leaders are compelled to change system processes to remain fiscally sound. Nurses benefit from this system approach that focuses on efficient practice grounded in quality care. These improvements are based on the Toyota production system principles of removing wasted time, movement, and resources.[23] Barnas and Adams[23] noted, however, that Lean processes are not enough, and the practices of gaining efficiency in all that is done need to be integrated into the culture throughout the organization.

Plan-do-study-act is the basis of Lean process changes and stems from W. Edwards Deming's ongoing improvement work on total quality management, with the driving focus on the concept that quality can always be better.[24] The individual and the system must continually work on improvement.[10] By involving bedside or direct care nurses in the total quality management process, they learn cause and effect while improving processes and improving care.[10]

Technology

Technology can either support or hinder the efficiency of a nurse. Extensive technology requirements associated with patient care can lead to nurse frustration and inefficiency.[25] There often are interruptions in a nurse's workflow and learning as new equipment is introduced. As noted by the National Academy of Medicine, innovations may benefit millions of patients, yet they often challenge nurses with complexity.[26] It also is noted that technology can support continual learning and create efficiencies for nurses.[26] Technology often is sought after for efficiency and to promote standardization of care. New technology can be disruptive to nurses who must change their processes due to the equipment or support systems. When technology is embraced and new processes are learned, the technology often is the more efficient answer to the provision of care. Nurses who are looking for a place of employment now explore the technology being used, the age of the technology, and the upgrade or replacement plans. New nurses also inquire what technology the organization has invested in to support the nursing staff in the organization. Some of the technologies are simple and focus on nursing efficiencies, such as phones or nursing call systems. Other technologies are more complex and when embraced can create efficiencies throughout the workday.[27]

Portable Communication Tools

There are support pieces of equipment that help nurses be more efficient. Research on the use of smartphones and effects on efficiency is in the early stages. More cost-effective phones do not have the ability to access the Internet yet save nurses travel time to desk or to hall phones to communicate. Some health care organizations have begun to use iPhones as a nurse's personal computer. These types of devices can be cost prohibitive for many organizations, limiting the opportunity for assessment. The more complex phones are minicomputers that are loaded with medical information. The technology creates an easy way to access evidence at the bedside as well as policy and procedural manuals, all while allowing for easier POC documentation. Several devices have the capability of being used for medication administration as well. A pocket device can be an efficient means of documentation, data retrieval, and overall management.[27]

Call Systems

Technology to aid nurses at the bedside is always evolving. Nurse call systems have become more creative and user-friendly. Technology advancements can now integrate the call system with the portable phones.[25] This technology decreases steps and helps the nursing team be more efficient. There are systems that can differentiate the types of calls between calls that are for the assistive personnel and those for the nursing staff. Decreasing interruptions is important as novice nurses establish their routine and create efficiencies.

Smart Pumps

The use of smart intravenous (IV) pumps creates efficiencies while supporting best evidence and safe practice. The novice nurse is supported by many factors by the smart IV pumps, such as medication dosing, educational references, and drug compatibility. Smart pumps are a safety tool because they place parameters on high-risk medications to avoid dosing errors. Evidence-based programs within the pumps save time by having references for dosing, indications, and interactions. The smart pump is an efficient system supporting safe patient care.[27]

Electronic Medical Record

The electronic medical record (EMR) is one of the most complex tools used in health care and serves as an efficiency tool guiding a nurse's practice.[28] Documenting at the POC is instrumental in efficiency of the EMR and improved outcomes. Creating this practice of POC documentation can quickly become a learned habit when practiced at the time of orientation and when new work flows are being developed. It is pivotal that preceptors engage in this practice as they orient the novice nurse. The EMR also provides other tools for time management beyond the documentation functions. Embracing the EMR and using the following tools within it are instrumental in gaining the available efficiencies.[26,27]

Decision support

Decision support systems are the tools embedded in the EMR. Decision support tools prompt nurses on practice decisions and are based on the best research evidence. Organizations build the support system within the routine documentation and workflow processes. Novice nurses learn as they are guided in their practice in an efficient manner with the support of decision support systems tools.[26] Decision support examples can include hospital initiatives, such as a sepsis care bundle or checklist. When certain triggers or indicators of impeding sepsis are noted, the system can send an alarm to the nurse for further investigation. These processes can be lifesaving as well as time saving. Tools that build nursing knowledge are viewed as an advantage when applied to care at the bedside.[26,27]

Nurses often are in the space of multitasking, and novice nurses are working on understanding the complexity of patients while being efficient in their practice. Having a system, such as the EMR, with decision support helps guide a nurse's critical thinking and can be a valuable resource. The system can identify that there could be upcoming patient issues and the EMR can trigger an alert. The alert can guide the nurse to begin nurse-driven protocols and seek out additional assistance.[26,27]

Nurse-driven protocols

Nurse-driven protocols allow nurses to practice at the full extent of their scope of practice.[27] The nurse can enact approved order sets that are based on decisions regarding certain patient criteria and presentation. Examples of nursing protocols are varied and include indwelling catheter removal, potassium replacement, or a ventilation weaning program. Protocols can be initiated by a nurse based on a patient's situation and a nurse's competency.

The large numbers of diverse protocols create efficiency by decreasing calls to physicians for orders as well as the potential to improve a patient's length of stay. Order sets also create consistency in patient care and allow for nurses to create an efficiency as how they deliver high-quality patient care. Order sets are built within the EMR and the care often is delivered within a nurse's work list.[27]

Work lists and to-do lists

Work lists and to-do lists live within most EMRs and are created to guide efficient work throughout a nurse's day. Most work lists can be created by nurses to support their daily routine and can be adjusted to meet the needs of the individual nurse. The work from protocols and decision support often is part of a work list or to-do list.[27]

Not all reminders are built into decision support because over-notifications can lead to alarm fatigue. Alarm fatigue is when systems over-alert and alarms are ignored.[27] It is important to have staff input as to which vital alarms are included and which are not. There also is the ability for individualization of the work lists as nurses strive to provide standardization to their lists. The list can include regulated care and focused organizational initiatives. This routine keeps nurses focused on important tasks while not having to write and rewrite paper lists on a daily basis. This focused approach creates efficiency in providing quality patient care during the day and at times of care transitions between shifts.[18,26,27]

FINAL THOUGHTS

Efficiencies for novice nurses are learned and gained through a systems approach as well as individually developed. Combined, there are tools and strategies that novice nurses acquire with the help of preceptors and mentors to become efficient members of a team and to successfully reach and function as an advanced beginner nurse. Through the tools and strategies described previously, nurses learn and grow to perform their skills at a highly efficient level and contribute to the overall organizational mission to support the triple aim. Both the personal tools and systems support structures are interconnected and facilitate safe, quality patient care. The nurse leader plays an important role to understand the support systems and to ensure that ongoing development for new nurses is encouraged and supported. The nurse leader is instrumental in the novice nurse transition to advanced beginner and to ultimately supporting the organization's quality, safety, and fiscal goals.

DISCLOSURE

The authors have nothing to disclose.

REFERENCES

1. Benner P. From novice to expert. Am J Nurs 1982;82:402–7.
2. Marshall ES, Broome ME. Transformational leadership in nursing. 2nd edition. New York: Springer Publishing Company; 2017. p. 63–80.

3. The IHI triple aim initiative. Institute for Healthcare Improvement. 2019. Available at: http://www.ihi.org/Engage/Initiatives/TripleAim/Pages/default.aspx. Accessed April 1, 2019.

4. Hendrix TJ. Optimization techniques: industrial production tools with application in nurse staffing efficiency research. Outcomes Manag 2003;7:194–7.

5. Huntington A, Gilmour J, Tuckett A, et al. Is anybody listening? A qualitative study of nurses' reflections on practice. J Clin Nurs 2011;20(9–10):1413–22.

6. Waterworth S. Time management strategies in nursing practice. J Adv Nurs 2003; 43:432–40.

7. Using logic models to bring together planning, evaluation, and action: logic model development guide. W. K. Kellogg Foundation; 2006. Available at: https://www.wkkf.org/resource-directory/resource/2006/02/wk-kellogg-foundation-logic-model-development-guide. Accessed April 1, 2019.

8. Shaw P, Abbott M, King TS. Preparation for practice in newly licensed registered nurses: a Mixed-Methods Descriptive Survey of Preceptors. J Nurses Prof Dev 2018;34:325–31.

9. Baumann A, Hunsberger M, Crea-Arsenio M, et al. Policy to practice: investment in transitioning new graduate nurses to the workplace. J Nurs Manag 2018;26: 373–81.

10. Marquis BL, Huston CJ. Socializing and educating staff in a learning organization. In: Leadership roles and management functions in nursing. 9th edition. Philadelphia: Wolters Kluwer; 2017. p. 407–49.

11. Kohtz C. Stack the odds in favor of newly licensed RNs. Nurs Manage 2016; 47:22–8.

12. Stone TE, Treloar AE. How did it get so late so soon?: tips and tricks for managing time. Nurs Health Sci 2015;17:409–11.

13. Kirkwood C. Why we are not getting enough sleep. Sci Am 2014. Available at: http://www.blogs.scientificamerica.com. Accessed May 1, 2019.

14. Weick KE, Sutcliffe K. Expectations and mindfulness. In: Managing the unexpected: resilient performance in an age of uncertainty. San Francisco (CA): Jossey-Bass; 2007. p. 23–42.

15. Bevins R, De Smet A. Making time management the organization's priority. McKinsey Quarterly 2013;1:26–41.

16. Bergman C, Shubert L. Interactive strategies: time management, prioritization, and delegation. Nurse Educ 2013;38:137–8.

17. Chan EA, Jones A, Wong K. The relationships between communication, care and time are intertwined: a narrative inquiry exploring the impact of time on registered nurses' work. J Adv Nurs 2012;69:2020–9.

18. The future of nursing leading change advancing health. Institute of Medicine; 2010. Available at: http://www.nationalacademies.org/hmd/Reports/2010/The-Future-of-Nursing-Leading-Change-Advancing-Health.aspx. Accessed April 15, 2019.

19. Cornell P, Townsend-Gervis M, Vardama J, et al. Improving situation awareness and patient outcomes through interdisciplinary rounding and structured communication. J Nurs Adm 2014;44(3):164–9.

20. Roussel L, Thomas P, Harris JL. Professional practice: a prototype linking nursing in interprofessional teams. In: Management and leadership for nursing administrators. 8th edition. Burlington (VT): Jones and Bartlett Learning; 2020. p. 45–53.

21. Kenney C. Transforming health care: Virginia mason medical center's pursuit of the perfect patient experience. New York: Productivity Press; 2011.

22. Lee JY, McFadden KL, Gowen CR. An exploratory analysis for lean and six sigma implementation in hospitals. Health Care Manage Rev 2018;43(3):182–92.
23. Barnas K, Adams E. Beyond heroes: a lean management system for healthcare. Appleton (WI): Jenkins Group; 2014.
24. Plan do study act. Institute for Healthcare Improvement; 2017. Available at: http://www.ihi.org/resources/Pages/Tools/PlanDoStudyActWorksheet.aspxlan do study act. Accessed April 3, 2019.
25. Zadvinskis IM, Garvey Smith J, Yen PY. Nurses' experience with health information technology: longitudinal qualitative study. JMIR Med Inform 2018;6(2):e38.
26. Best care at lower cost: the path to continuously leaning healthcare in America. Institute of Medicine; 2012. Available at: http://www.nationalacademies.org/hmd/Reports/2012/Best-Care-at-Lower-Cost-The-Path-to-Continuously-Learning-Health-Care-in-America.aspx. Accessed April 30, 2019.
27. McGonigle D, Mastrian KG. Translational research: generating evidence for practice. In: Nursing informatics and the foundation of knowledge. Burlington (VT): Jones and Bartlett Learning; 2018. p. 495–506.
28. O'Brien A, Weaver C, Settergren T, et al. EHR documentation. Nurs Adm Q 2015; 39(4):333–9.

An Interprofessional Model with Registered Nurses for Outpatient Care

Mary Alyce Nelson, DNP, RN

KEYWORDS

- Interprofessional • Mental illness • Outpatient • Registered nurse • Nurse • RN
- Mental health

KEY POINTS

- Mental illness is an area of concern to nurses.
- Registered nurses (RNs) have an opportunity and obligation to expand roles and positively affect outpatient mental health care.
- A new model titled the "mental health outpatient with nurses interprofessional team (MONIT) model is proposed to expand the role of RNs.
- The MONIT model can improve accessibility and quality of outpatient mental health care.

INTRODUCTION

Registered nurses (RNs) have an opportunity and obligation to expand roles and positively affect outpatient mental health care in the United States. In 2016, an estimated 44.7 million adults in the United States reported experiencing a mental illness.[1] Mental illness causes more disability in industrialized nations than other chronic illnesses including cancer and heart disease.[2] Mental illness is the tenth leading cause of death in the United States.[3] In 2016, one-third of people diagnosed with mental illness did not receive treatment.[1] Identified barriers to treatment include lack of insurance coverage, lack of affordable care, and lack of available treatment providers.[4] People who live in rural areas are especially challenged due to limited access to mental health care due to a shortage of mental health professionals and psychiatrists.[5] One study reported that two-thirds of primary care physicians claimed that they could not obtain psychiatric referrals for their clients.[6] Proposed solutions to the shortage of mental health providers include service integration, workforce training, and new treatment models.[7] A new mental health outpatient with nurses interprofessional team (MONIT) model is a potential solution that will improve access and quality of outpatient care for people experiencing mental illness.

College of Nursing, The Pennsylvania State University, 206D Nursing Sciences Building, University Park, PA 16802, USA
E-mail address: mun138@psu.edu

Nurs Clin N Am 55 (2020) 51–60
https://doi.org/10.1016/j.cnur.2019.10.005
0029-6465/20/© 2019 Elsevier Inc. All rights reserved.

nursing.theclinics.com

SIGNIFICANCE TO NURSING PRACTICE

Mental illness is an issue with great significance to RNs working in all areas of nursing. Mental illness affects the lives of many individuals, and 44.7 million Americans reported having a diagnosis of mental illness in 2016.[1] Serious mental illness leads to significant impairment that affects quality and life and ability to function independently for 13.6 million Americans.[8] Timely, efficient, and effective care for mental disorders is needed, but access to mental health treatment is limited.[5] Approximately one-third of people diagnosed with mental illness were unable to access care in 2016.[1]

There are serious consequences to untreated mental illness. Suicide can result when treatment is not readily available or is ineffective, and it is the tenth leading cause of death in the United States.[3] Adults between ages 45 and 54 years have the highest suicide rate (19.72), and the overall age-adjusted suicide rate is 13.2 per 100,00 individuals.[3] Individuals diagnosed with mental illness such as borderline personality disorder, depression, bipolar disorder, and opioid use with depression have rates of suicide that are estimated at 10 times greater than the general population.[9] Suicide is not the only serious consequence of mental illness. People diagnosed with mental illness suffer from comorbid health conditions such as asthma, diabetes, high blood pressure, cardiac disease, and stroke.[10] In addition, life expectancies of individuals who struggle with severe mental illness are approximately 10 years less than the general population.[10]

Mental illness and related disorders in the United States result in large financial burden. The causes of high cost include loss of income due to unemployment, expenses for supportive programs, medical charges for psychiatric care, and treatment of comorbid medical conditions.[10,11] It is estimated that the fiscal burden in the United States caused by major depression alone increased by 21.5% from $173.2 billion in 2005 to $210.5 billion in 2010.[11] Mental disorders caused the highest overall spending in 2013, with spending rates exceeding trauma, heart conditions, and pulmonary conditions.[12]

Individuals with mental illness incur high costs due to use of emergency services and inpatient hospitalizations.[13] Rates of emergency room visits for mental health reasons such as anxiety, depression, bipolar disorder, and substance abuse increased by 44.1%, whereas visits for suicidal ideation increased by 44.6% between 2006 and 2014.[14] Individuals experiencing mental health crises are more likely to be hospitalized when they receive care in emergency departments rather than receiving care from community mental health providers.[15] Emergency providers seek inpatient hospitalization when individuals pose a risk of harm to self or others.[16] Emergency hospitalization can be diverted by quality community mental health services that are readily accessible to provide immediate intervention and stabilization of symptoms.[5] Unfortunately, 77% of counties in the United States have inadequate numbers of psychiatrists and other mental health professionals to meet the demand for services.[5]

RNs can be instrumental in finding solutions for health care provider shortages, improving management of patient mental health care, and decreasing the economic burden of mental illness.[17] The addition of RNs to interprofessional outpatient mental health teams will allow for more efficient and holistic care management.[1] Team-based models and the role of the RN have mainly been studied in primary and specialty care settings. Researchers identify positive outcomes when RNs are included as part of an integrated team model in general health settings.[18–21] Researchers also identify positive outcomes when RNs are added as care coordinators in specialty outpatient offices that address diabetes[22] and hypertension.[23,24] Substance Abuse and Mental Health Services Administration[25] recommends the addition of RNs to outpatient models to increase access and quality of care. There is a gap in the literature regarding research that is specifically focused on adding RNs to interprofessional teams in the specialty area of mental health.

One proposed solution to the shortage of mental health treatment involves integration of physical and mental health services. Most of the research in this area focuses on integrating mental health services into primary care settings, and this shows some success in the medical home model.[26] Sklar and colleagues[20] found that adding behavioral health specialists to address mental health concerns in primary care outpatient settings increases the recovery success of mental health clients. Another study reported positive outcomes when interprofessional team services were added at several mental health care clinics in the Veterans Administration system.[27] Some care models included RNs in the team, but effectiveness related to the specific professional team members was not studied.

Alternatives to treatment delivered at outpatient mental health clinics have also been proposed.[1] Traditional mental health treatment centers are stand-alone clinics that solely offer behavioral health services.[1] Clients meet individually with specific providers to target precise needs, such as a psychiatrist for medication evaluations, case managers for communications with outside services, and therapists for counseling. A patient may require several different visits at the same clinic with different providers over a period of a few months. An interprofessional model that involves a team approach where all members could address most patient care needs in one visit can help to decrease the need for multiple appointments and subsequently improve treatment accessibility for more individuals.[28] Some experts suggest that the addition of RNs to interprofessional outpatient mental health teams will allow for more efficient care management, because the scope of practice encompasses physical as well as behavioral health.[1]

WHY NURSES MUST BE INVOLVED IN OUTPATIENT TREATMENT OF MENTAL ILLNESS

RNs are academically prepared to provide care to individuals with mental illness. RNs have contact with individuals with mental illness in all areas of nursing practice, and nurses must have sufficient knowledge of mental health concepts. The Essentials of Baccalaureate Education for Professional Nursing Practice authored by the American Association of Colleges of Education[29] calls for a solid knowledge base in liberal education that includes aspects of mental health such as psychology, spirituality, and cultural concerns. Quality care and patient safety addressed in Essential II are current concerns in the area of outpatient mental health care. Consideration of health care and economics that are current issues in mental health care are addressed in Essential V, and the importance of interprofessional communication and collaboration is highlighted in Essential VI. Finally, Essential IX addresses that the RN with a bachelor's degree is prepared to practice with patients of all ages and across various health care environments.[29] Of course, one important practice environment includes the area of mental health.

Professional nurses have a responsibility to provide care to all individuals in need of care, and the need is great in the area of mental health. The American Nurses Association has established professional Nursing's Scope and Standards of Practice to define and describe nursing practice.[30] The scope, or definition of nursing practice, includes RNs who are licensed by state entities who practice in various environments where care is necessary. Nurses use knowledge based on education, experiences, and the needs of the population served. Nursing practice can adapt based on changing societal requirements as dictated by the obligation to provide care.[30] Based on this definition and the current shortage of timely and efficient outpatient mental health care, it is apparent that nurses have a duty to expand practice roles in order to provide better care to individuals with mental illness.

Standards of professional nursing practice include assessment, diagnosis, outcomes identification, planning, implementation, coordination of care, health teaching and health promotion, and evaluation.[30] Nurses can have great impact through application of these standards to mental health care. RNs practicing at the full scope of practice allowed by state licensing boards can effectively assess, treat, and coordinate care for individuals experiencing mental health concerns in all practice settings. Specifically, nurses practicing in expanded roles in mental health outpatient settings can have a great impact on quality and accessibility of care.

Hildegard Peplau's Framework for Psychodynamic Nursing[31] views nursing as an interpersonal process and places great emphasis on the importance of the nurse–patient relationship. There are 4 specific and related phases of the nurse–patient relationship, including orientation, identification, exploitation, and resolution. There are specific tasks in each phase as well as situational roles demanded of the nurse. Some roles include teacher, counselor, surrogate, technical expert, and others.[31] The nurse initially assists the patient to identify and recognize the need for help. The patient is then guided by the nurse in further exploring and working toward mutually identified outcomes and ultimate problem resolution. Peplau also emphasizes that nurses must engage in interpersonal relationships in all areas of nursing.[31]

CURRENT EVIDENCE: NURSES ON INTERPROFESSIONAL TEAMS ADDRESSING MENTAL HEALTH ISSUES

Past research studies focusing on interprofessional models of treatment of clients with mental illness have been conducted in various settings, and the design of the models are varied. All of the studies included in this review addresses interprofessional teams in some manner. For purposes of this review, the information is organized as follows:

1. Interprofessional teams in primary health care settings
   a. Models with RN management
   b. Models developed due to government initiatives
   c. Study focused on supportive structure of model
2. Interprofessional teams in outpatient clinics that deliver only mental health care
3. The RN role in interprofessional teams in outpatient mental health settings
4. Interprofessional teams addressing mental illness in mental health outpatient clinics

Interprofessional Teams in Primary Health Care Settings

Previous research about interprofessional teams that include nurses focuses primarily on the improvement of both mental illness and chronic physical illness.[20,26,32–37] Some studies focus on introducing new models of care that involve RN management of both mental and chronic physical health symptoms.[32–35] Most of these studies focus on patients who were treated in an outpatient primary care setting,[32,33,35] and one study involves patients who were treated in a mental health clinic.[34] RNs have key roles as case/care managers and are responsible for coordination of care.[32–35] The nursing role functions include assessment of physical symptoms, mental health symptoms, counseling, and communication through team meetings.[32,34,35,38] The models include regular visits to assess physical and mental health symptoms.[32,34,35,38] RNs are trained to act as counselors in order to be adept at assisting with physical and mental health symptoms.[32,34,35,38] Nurses have specific guidelines to follow to guide interventions and provide alerts when referral or acute intervention from a physician or other team member is indicated.[34,35,38] RNs are also educated about coaching patients through the use of cognitive and behavioral techniques such as motivational interviewing to encourage positive health behaviors.[32,34,35,38] Treatment teams meet regularly to collaborate on the plan of treatment, discuss progress, and make treatment decisions.[32,34,35]

Some studies involve teams treating mental health and physical symptoms investigated team models that were developed secondary to government initiatives.[20,26,36] Two studies refer to the medical home model design that addresses treatment of mental illness and physical disease, but service delivery models vary. One study reflects that the primary care team treats both physical and mental health needs, and specialty mental health providers are communicated with on a regular basis for care coordination purposes.[26] Another approach is the establishment of a joint administrative and clinical unit to promote information sharing and address educational needs of staff.[20] RN care coordinators and behavioral health consultants are employed to address mental health needs.[20] Goldstein[36] concludes that fully integrated care requires a team of full-time psychiatrist, care coordinators, and mental health professionals who are located in the same location as primary care.

Fortney and colleagues[37] address teams designed to treat physical and mental illness focused on the need to provide a well-defined and supportive structure to facilitate the adoption of interprofessional teams. Supportive mentoring and leadership structures can help with the successful development, implementation, and success of interprofessional team models. An evidence-based quality improvement framework can provide a guiding structure and continuous feedback during the planning phases of a collaborative team care model.[37]

Interprofessional Teams in Outpatient Clinics that Deliver Mental Health Care

Only 3 studies in this review describe interprofessional teams implemented in outpatient clinics that solely deliver mental health care.[27,28,39] The models emphasize communication between team members such as RNs, psychologists, psychiatrists, social workers, recreational therapists, mental health counselors, and others. Regular and well-structured treatment team meetings are held to review progress and establish treatment plans.[27,28] The team may also participate in daily huddles to review cases of patients who are scheduled for visits, identify patients with acute needs, and review operational issues.[27] Patient input on treatment planning and presence at team meetings is required at established time intervals to develop and evaluate progress toward goals.[28]

Two of the three studies that focus on interprofessional teams in outpatient clinics are conducted in mental health clinics and involve provision of direct care.[27,28] The third study focuses on an interprofessional practice-based research network (PBRN) to promote mentoring, support, and application of evidence-based research for providers of integrated mental health services.[39] The PBRN was found to support collaboration between leaders in the mental health community, leaders from 3 mental health agencies, and experts from an academic partner.[39] The specific interprofessional team model that provided direct service to outpatients is not described.

The Role of Registered Nurses in Interprofessional Teams in Outpatient Mental Health Settings

The National Council Medical Director Institute[5] calls for all mental health clinicians to practice at the full scope allowed by licensure. Barry and colleagues[27] reflect that, when allowed to exercise full scope of practice, RNs can fill care management roles that allow other team members to also function at their highest practice levels and that they are important members of interprofessional teams designed to treat clients with mental illness. Several models in this review specifically include RNs in key roles such as direct care provider, case manager, or care coordinators.[20,32,34,35,38] In these models, RNs are expected to assess and treat patients, make care decisions, and communicate with other interprofessional team members. The 2 articles that were completed in mental health clinics report that RNs are included, although the specific role of the nurse is not identified.[27,28] There is a gap in the literature related to the role of the RN on interprofessional teams in mental health settings.

THE MENTAL HEALTH OUTPATIENT WITH NURSE INTERPROFESSIONAL TEAM MODEL

A new model titled the "mental health outpatient with nurses interprofessional team" model is proposed to expand the role of RNs working in coordination with a team of mental health professionals (Nelson MA. Implementing an innovative interprofessional mental health outpatient model with nurses to improve care [Unpublished manuscript; DNP Project]. 2019. Available at: https://scholarsphere.psu.edu/concern/generic_works/fj6731449q.Accessed May 20, 2019). The MONIT model replaces the traditional model of care that involves separate appointments with various team members. The model expands all team member capabilities so that clients do not need to make multiple appointments to have their needs met. This increases access to care by freeing up appointment slots, and clients who are encountering stressful situations are able to make appointments. All team members are trained to assist clients who are experiencing distress, and this helps to decrease the number of clients using costly emergency room care and inpatient hospitalization. **Fig. 1** depicts the MONIT model.

The MONIT model expands the role of the RN to include medication management. Nursing visits will replace some routine medication management visits with the psychiatrist to assess medication efficacy. The nurse may use an electronic health record

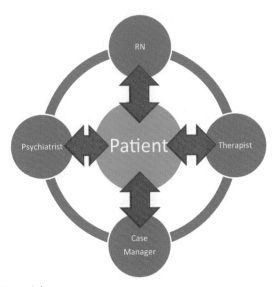

Fig. 1. The MONIT model.

template designed in collaboration with medical staff. Some of the areas of assessment include evaluation of vital signs, medication efficacy, evaluation of side effects, compliance, need for refills, etc. It would also be important to evaluate patient perception of medication efficacy and comfort level with the medication. The nurse could also provide ongoing medication education during the visit. **Box1** includes some specific questions that can be added to a medication management visit.

A key feature of the MONIT model involves the use of team huddles designed to increase communication between team members. During the huddle, clients who are on the daily schedule are discussed, and team members communicate about clients who have called with any issues or problems. Team members collaborate to best address patient needs and service coordination. Clients who are experiencing immediate problems may be scheduled open appointments with the team member who can best address individual needs. One example of this might be a client who is complaining of medication side effects that can be addressed by an RN rather than a psychiatrist.

Joanne Duffy's Quality Caring Model[40] is used to structure the MONIT model. The major proposition of the Quality Caring Model is that caring relationships support and influence the attainment of positive health outcomes for clients, families, communities, health care providers, and health care systems. The 4 main concepts of the model include (1) humans in relationships, (2) relationship-centered professional encounters, (3) clients and families who feel cared for, and (4) self-advancing systems.[40]

The Quality Caring Model[40] offers a framework that, when applied to MONIT model, purposes structure, process, and outcomes. The structure of the model includes participants who will be the clinic outpatients and their family members; nurses and other interprofessional team members; and other systems that could include health clinics, communities, and area health centers. The process will be relationship centered and will involve caring and collaborative communications among clients as well as interprofessional team members. The outcomes encompass measures that reflect the patient, provider, and the system. This model can be specifically applied to outcomes that will focus on the patient, such as symptom improvement, appointment compliance, access, and use of services.

More specifically, the framework is applied to the MONIT model to define the team member roles and functions. The traditional outpatient team model involves individual interactions with mental health professionals in order to meet specific needs, and clients might have to visit the clinic several times a month to meet with various professionals. The RN role in the traditional model is to deal with physical health concerns or

---

Box 1
Questions for registered nurses to include in medication management visit

What medications are currently prescribed?

Are you taking all of your medications as prescribed? RN should check medicine bottles to confirm.

Are you taking any over-the-counter medications? Any supplements or herbal supplements?

Have you experienced any problems related to your medications?

Are your medications helping or not helping? Please explain.

Are you requesting any changes to your medications? If yes, please explain.

Do you need any refills? RN should check medicine bottles to confirm.

to coordinate care with physical health providers. The MONIT model is intended to expand the role of the RN and includes mental health assessment, planning, and interventions. RNs participate with other team members in evaluating and revising mental health care plans. In addition, other team members are intended to experience expansion of roles. The intent of the model is to train team members to deal with multiple patient needs in order to improve efficiency of care and decrease the number of clinic visits and subsequently increase availability of open appointments. Communication between team members is projected to increase during huddles and treatment team meetings. These meetings are structured to enable early identification of clients who may be decompensating to allow for better symptom management. Also, all team members are trained to intervene in crisis situations, and this is projected to decrease emergency room visits and inpatient hospitalizations.

SUMMARY

RNs are currently in a key position to positively influence mental health treatment. RNs who are practicing in expanded roles can be valuable members of interprofessional teams in the outpatient mental health setting. The MONIT model provides a structured approach to mental health treatment in which RNs can practice at the full scope allowed by licensure. Nurses in all practice areas come in contact with individuals with mental health issues, and all RNs have an obligation to improve quality and access to care for individuals experiencing mental illness.

REFERENCES

1. Substance Abuse and Mental Health Services Administration. Key substance use and mental health indicators in the United States: Results from the 2016 national survey on drug use and health. 2017. Available at: https://www.samhsa.gov/data/sites/default/files/NSDUH-FFR1-2016/NSDUH-FFR1-2016.htm. Accessed April 14, 2019.
2. Vigo D, Thornicroft G, Atun A. Estimating the true global burden of mental illness. Lancet 2016;3(2):171–8.
3. Centers for Disease Control and Prevention. Ten leading causes of death and injury. Available at: https://www.cdc.gov/injury/wisqars/LeadingCauses.html. Accessed May 27, 2019.
4. Mental Health America. Mental health in America: access to care data. Available at: http://www.mentalhealthamerica.net/issues/mental-health-america-access-care-data. Accessed April 14, 2019.
5. National Council Medical Director Institute. The psychiatric shortage: causes and solutions(Report No. BH365). Available at: https://www.thenationalcouncil.org/wp-content/uploads/2017/03/Psychiatric-Shortage_National-Council-.pdf. Accessed May 27, 2019.
6. Roll JM, Kennedy J, Tran M, et al. Disparities in unmet need for mental health services in the United States, 1997-2010. Psychiatr Serv 2013;64:80–2. https://doi.org/10.1176/appi.Ps.201200071.
7. Knickman J, Krishnan KRR, Pincus HA, et al. Improving access to effective care for people who have mental health and substance use disorders [Discussion Paper]. Vital Directions for Health and Health Care Series. Available at: https://nam.edu/wp-content/uploads/2016/09/improving-access-to-effective-care-for-people-who-have-mentalhealth-and-substance-use-disorders.pdf. Accessed May 24, 2019.

8. National Institutes of Health. Serious mental illness among adults. Available at: https://www.nimh.nih.gov/health/statistics/prevalence/serious-mental-illness-smi-among-us-adults.shtml. Accessed May 24, 2019.

9. Chesney E, Goodwin GM, Fazel S. Risks of all-cause and suicide mortality in mental disorders: a meta-review. World Psychiatry 2014;13:153–60.

10. Walker ER, McGee RE, Druss BG. Mortality in mental disorders and global disease burden implications: A systematic review and meta-analysis. JAMA Psychiatry 2015;72(4):334–41.

11. Greenberg PE, Fournier A, Sisitsky T, et al. The economic burden of adults with major depressive disorder in the United States (2005 and 2010). J ClinPsychiatry 2015;76(2):155.

12. Roehrig C. Mental disorders top the list of the most costly conditions in the United States: $201 billion. HealthAff (Millwood) 2016;35(6):1130–5.

13. de Oliveira C, Cheng J, Vigod S, et al. Clients with high mental health costs incur over 30 percent more costs than other high-cost clients. HealthAff (Millwood) 2016;35(1):36.

14. Agency for Healthcare Review and Quality (AHRQ). Healthcare cost and utilization project: Statistical brief #277. Available at: https://www.hcup-us.ahrq.gov/reports/statbriefs/sb227-Emergency-Department-Visit-Trends.jsp. Accessed March 18, 2019.

15. Owens P, Mutter R, Stocks C. Mental health and substance-abuse related emergency department visits among adults, 2007. HCUP Statistical Brief #92. Available at: https://www.hcup-us.ahrq.gov/reports/statbriefs/sb92.pdf. Accessed May 27, 2019.

16. Pennsylvania Mental Health Procedures Act. Chapter 5100, Sections 5100.71-5100.86. 1996.

17. Rutherford MM. Enhanced RN role in behavioral health care: an untapped resource. Nurs Econ 2017;35:88–95.

18. Ku L, Frogner BK, Steinmetz E, et al. Community health centers employ diverse staffing patterns, which can provide productivity lessons for medical practices. Health Aff (Millwood) 2015;34(1):95–103.

19. Pittman P, Forrest E. The changing roles of registered nurses in pioneer accountable care organizations. NursOutlook 2015;63(5):554–65.

20. Sklar M, Aarons GA, O'Connell M, et al. Mental health recovery in the patient-centered medical home. Am J PublicHealth 2015;105(9):1926–34.

21. Stewart KR, Stewart GL, Lampman M, et al. Implications of the patient-centered medical home for nursing practice. J Nurs Adm 2015;45(11):569–74.

22. Myers JM. Interprofessional team management: partnering to optimize outcomes in diabetes. J NursePrac 2017;13(3):e147–50.

23. Biernacki PJ, Champagne MT, Peng S, et al. Transformation of Care: Integrating the registered nurse care coordinator into the patient-centered medical home. PopulHealthManag 2015;18:330–6.

24. Ehrlich C, Kendall E, St John W. How does care coordination provided by registered nurses "fit" within that organisational processes and professional relationships in the general practice context? Collegian 2013;20(3):127.

25. Substance Abuse and Mental Health Services Administration. Role of nurses in home health and integrated settings. Available at: https://integration.samhsa.gov/about-us/Nurses_role_in_integrated_care_slides.pdf. Accessed May 27, 2019.

26. Domino ME, Kilany M, Wells R, et al. Through the looking glass: estimating effects of medical homes for people with severe mental illness. HealthServ Res 2017; 52(5):1858–80.

27. Barry CN, Abraham KM, Weaver KR, et al. Innovating team-based outpatient mental health care in the veterans' health administration: Staff-perceived benefits and challenges to pilot implementation of the behavioral health interdisciplinary program (BHIP). Psychol Serv 2016;13(2):148–55.

28. Tippin GK, Maranzan A, Mountain MA. Client outcomes associated with interprofessional care in a community mental health outpatient program. Can J Commun-MentHealth 2016;35(3):83–96.

29. American Association of Colleges of Nursing (AACN). The essentials of baccalaureate education for professional nursing practice. Available at: https://www.aacnnursing.org/Education-Resources/AACN-Essentials. Accessed May 27, 2019.

30. American Nurses Association. Nursing: scope and standards of practice. Silver Spring (MD): American Nurses Association; 2015.

31. Peplau HE. Interpersonalrelations in nursing: a conceptual frame of reference for psychodynamic nursing. New York: Springer; 1991.

32. Bekelman DB, Hooker S, Nowels CT, et al. Feasibility and acceptability of a collaborative care intervention to improve symptoms and quality of life in chronic heart failure: mixed methods pilot trial. J Palliat Med 2014;17(2):145–51.

33. Morgan MAJ, Coates MJ, Dunbar JA, et al. The TrueBlue model of collaborative care using practice nurses as case managers for depression alongside diabetes or heart disease: a randomised trial. BMJ Open 2013;3(1):e002171.

34. Chwastiak LA, Luongo M, Russo J, et al. Use of a mental health center collaborative care team to improve diabetes care and outcomes for patients with psychosis. Psychiatr Serv 2018;69(3):349–52.

35. Katon WJ, Lin EHB, Von Korff M, et al. Collaborative care for clients with depression and chronic illnesses. N Engl J Med 2010;363(27):2611–20.

36. Goldstein EV. Integrating mental and physical health care for low-income Americans: Assessing a federal program's impact. Healthcare (Basel) 2017;5(3):32.

37. Fortney J, Enderle M, McDougall S, et al. Implementation outcomes of evidence-based quality improvement for depression in VA community based outpatient clinics. Implement Sci 2013;7(1):30–6.

38. Morgan S, Pullon S, McKinlay E. Observation of interprofessional collaborative practice in primary care teams: An integrative literature review. Int J Nurs Stud 2015;52(7):1217–30.

39. Kelly EL, Davis L, Brekke JS. PBRN findings: integrated care for individuals with serious mental illnesses. Psychiatr Serv 2015;66(11):1253.

40. Duffy JR. Quality caring in nursing and health systems: implications for clinicians, educators, and leaders. 2nd edition. New York: Springer Pub; 2013.

Developing Nurses Through Mentoring

It Starts in Nursing Education

Michael M. Evans, PhD, MSEd, RN, ACNS, CMSRN, CNE[a,*],
Kaléi Kowalchik[a], Kiernan Riley, BSN, RN[b], Lucy Adams[a]

KEYWORDS

- Mentoring • Benner • Professional development • Professional socialization
- Early socialization • Undergraduate nursing student • Faculty

KEY POINTS

- Faculty mentoring can enhance undergraduate student learning outside of the classroom and prepare them to be future leaders in the nursing profession.
- Faculty mentoring can provide students with cocurricular activities that they may not otherwise gain exposure to and help socialize them to various realms of nursing.
- The intrinsic and extrinsic value of faculty mentoring makes the added work of student mentoring invaluable.

In a time of a critical nursing shortage of not only bedside nurses but also advanced practice nurses, including nurse practitioners, researchers, and nurse educators, it is essential that experienced nurses share their expertise with novice learners to ensure the future success of the nursing profession. Currently in the United States, many hospitals are unable to fill up to 20% of their nursing positions.[1] Furthermore, the Bureau of Labor Statistics estimates that by 2024 there will be a need to fill more than 500,000 open nursing positions.[1] It is every nurse's responsibility to mentor and guide novice nurses, regardless of the setting, but nurse faculty can play a special role in helping to develop the next generation of nurse leaders through early socialization to the profession and specialty roles.[2,3] Therefore, the purpose of this article is to describe ways that nurse faculty can guide and mentor undergraduate and graduate nursing students to various nursing roles through early socialization to these roles to better prepare them to be future leaders in the nursing profession.

Mentorship in the nursing profession is a professional obligation and pivotal construct dedicated to bettering the future of nursing practice and clinical education.

[a] College of Nursing, The Pennsylvania State University, Scranton Campus, Dawson Room 111, 120 Ridge View Drive, Dunmore, PA 18512, USA; [b] College of Nursing, The Pennsylvania State University, University Park Campus, Nursing Sciences Building, Office 315H, 269 E. College Avenue, State College, PA 16802, USA
* Corresponding author.
E-mail address: mme124@psu.edu

Nurs Clin N Am 55 (2020) 61–69
https://doi.org/10.1016/j.cnur.2019.10.006
0029-6465/20/© 2019 Elsevier Inc. All rights reserved.

As the nurse transitions through Patricia Benner's 5 Stages of Clinical Competence, novice, advanced beginner, competent, proficient, and expert, mentorship guides the nurse at any stage of his/her progression, allowing the individual to develop skills to practice in their field. As the expert guides their mentoring novice throughout these multiple stages of the clinical and educational development, the mentor increases in his/her competence regarding knowledge of mentoring practices in the workplace, evaluating the novice, identifying needs, supporting the learning processes and goal orientation in mentoring, and providing constructive feedback. Professional socialization will allow the mentee to create a structured foundation of knowledge, skills, and values of the profession, which will develop as he or she progresses throughout the 5 Stages of Clinical Competence.[4]

In the nursing field, mentorship builds skills, knowledge, and core values of the profession. As the student builds his or her academic and professional career from novice to expert, he or she will partake in multiple mentoring relationships, which will allow them to develop the necessary abilities to connect with the profession. Mentorship is interconnected throughout an individual's growth in their nursing profession: multiple professional relationships can exist and will motivate the student and novice nurse to become more competent care providers in their area of work. The continuous connections that are built between mentors and mentees then improve the novice's ability to better deal with negative feelings, which ultimately increases their levels of self-esteem, confidence, comfort, and competence with professional skills.[5]

This mentoring relationship can and should develop during one's nursing education. Nursing faculty has a unique role with the ability to work individually and in teams with undergraduate and graduate nursing students, depending on their teaching and advising responsibilities. Nursing faculty members are expected to prepare graduates to enter an increasingly complex profession while also providing service, conducting research, maintaining clinical skills, and enhancing their teaching.[6] It is through these areas of conducting research, maintaining clinical expertise, and professional development opportunities whereby faculty can enhance a student's education outside of the classroom and provide them with cocurricular experiences that will not only enhance their educational experience but also provide them with socialization to areas of nursing that they may not otherwise get exposure to.[7] This exposure can lead students to gain interest in a new area of nursing and even consider exploring further education in this area as well as prepare them for future mentoring relationships in their field of choice.[8] In the following paragraphs, a description of how to work with students on a daily to weekly basis to help them acclimate into the nursing profession and provide them with experiences that will enhance their education and help prepare them as future leaders of the profession is provided. In addition, vignettes (Appendices 1–3) are provided by a few mentored students to outline how they value the mentoring experience.

IMPLEMENTATION OF A FACULTY LED MENTORING PROGRAM

The later discussion outlines steps that faculty can take to implement a mentoring program. This listed process is not all inclusive, but it can serve as a guide for faculty to use when implementing their own mentoring program with students.

Identification of Mentees

The first step in implementing a nursing faculty–led mentoring program is to identify students who would be interested in "extra" cocurricular nursing-related experiences. Obviously, not all students are interested or able to partake in such experiences, nor will a faculty member be able to mentor all students by himself or herself. It is critical that all faculty buys into the importance of mentoring students because it would be impossible for 1 faculty member to have the time and expertise to help all interested students.

To find interested students, the faculty member should announce openings for research team positions or an opportunity for students to shadow during the faculty's clinical work during a honor's meetings or class. Faculty can also send out e-mails to nursing students in various cohorts, describing what they are looking for in a team member. It is important to mentor 1 student from each year in the nursing program (freshman, sophomore, junior, and senior student). Mentoring students with various educational backgrounds is beneficial for several reasons. First, freshmen and sophomores can learn by just attending weekly team research meetings and partaking in small tasks, such as finding relevant research on a research topic, helping with formatting a manuscript to a specific referencing style, and/or helping with the development and writing of a manuscript or poster. Second, it allows more experienced students on the team (junior and senior undergraduate students and graduate students) to mentor the novice members. If more students show an interest than you are able to mentor, meet with all of them for a brief interview to find a student who "fits" best with your interest area or areas. After selecting the student or students to join the research team, try to work with the other students to find other identifiable mentors to connect with.

Implementation of Mentoring Program

It is critical to have clear expectations and guidelines when developing a mentoring program with students. As a faculty member, you cannot expect an 18-year-old student to be as disciplined, excited, or knowledgeable about a project as you, the expert, are. However, it is reasonable to expect a mentee to work autonomously when possible, use resources available to them (APA manual, readings provided to him or her, and each other), and to ask questions when he or she does not understand something. Faculty members can look at their mentoring program of students through the lens of Patricia Benner's theory of novice to expert. Faculty should meet students/mentees where they are and guide them through the various stages of Benner's theory; it is important to remember that this takes time and patience.[9] One should expect mistakes: you are working with students, not colleagues, who make mistakes also, but just not as frequently. Faculty must help students overcome these errors and not become discouraged. Faculty should provide fair constructive feedback to the student mentees. It is okay to be critical when necessary and nurture the student when needed, and knowing when to do which is just as crucial and is something that is perceived differently with each student based on his/her personality.

After identifying a group of mentees, it is important to set the expectation of regular contact. It is recommended to hold weekly research/team meetings around their school schedule, not your schedule. Although you may rather meet at 9 AM, that may not work for the team. Sometimes the meeting time may not be the most ideal time but will work for everyone else on the team, which is most important. To identify a time to meet, you can use a doodle poll at the start of each semester and select the day/time with the most responses to be chosen for the meeting. This task is something that can easily be delegated to a "junior" team member.

During the meeting, it is critical to clear the calendar for the meeting and stay focused on tasks that need attention during this time. It is recommended to hold 1-hour meetings weekly during the academic year and as needed over the summer months. During these 1-hour meetings, have an agenda sent out before the meeting so that everyone comes to the meeting prepared. The meetings are only attended by team members, unless a guest is invited for a special reason, for example, the need for statistical expertise. Start each meeting with a 5- to 10-minute round robin whereby each mentee can ask any questions related to school or other issues that he or she may be having at the time. This round robin is critical because it shows that you, as the leader, care about each member as an individual and are willing to listen to their concerns and help them problem solve concerns that he or she may be having. Following this, each team member has items listed under an agenda to provide updates on. As with any project, the amount of time each member needs to discuss their items varies, and thus, the amount of time dedicated to each mentee varies with each meeting. For example, if someone is preparing a poster for a conference, he or she may get more time to display their poster for editing purposes than someone who is just starting the literature review for a project.

Types of Mentoring Experiences

The types of mentoring experiences that you make available to students will vary based on your expertise, job responsibilities, and mentees. If you are not prepared as a researcher and are clinical faculty, you may offer to have a student or two shadow you while you are working in the clinical setting. Students can shadow faculty in a variety of clinical experiences that they may not otherwise gain experience, such as nursing supervision, hospice, home health, nurse practitioner practice, nursing administration, and more. These experiences are invaluable for students because they gain exposure to a variety of nursing experience that they may not otherwise gain experience in. They get to learn from an expert and are provided with appropriate role modeling in the clinical setting, which they may not always get during their routine clinical experiences. They also benefit from one-on-one time with their mentor and get the personal attention that may be lacking during routine clinical experiences during their schooling.

During these experiences, students/mentees can learn and enhance their clinical reasoning and judgment skills while working within a close one-on-one environment. In addition, students gain valuable communication skills by watching and participating in interactions with a mentor. For an enriching learning experience to occur, it is critical that the mentee feels comfortable talking with their mentor, and one can influence this by treating him or her as a colleague and not a student during these experiences. A collegial relationship also helps the student "up their game" and realize that you have high expectations for him or her.

Another avenue of mentoring experience that can be provided to students is in the research realm. Research projects typically revolve around the mentor's areas of interest, but you can also dabble in other areas that mentees are interested in and provide methodological support rather than content expertise. It is during a project like this that you may need to consult outside expertise and invite others to the meetings. It is important to relinquish lead authorship when mentoring students and let them take the lead. It can be difficult to do, but if they are prepared, you just might be surprised at how well they do. It is critical to keep your mentees involved in other research events. For example, forward e-mails to mentees for outside research opportunities: this can include serving on boards, such as the campus academic integrity and research committees, completing research and evidence-based practice modules, attendance at hospital based grand round events, campus lunch and learn talks, weekly nursing research seminars that only graduate students typically attend as part of their curriculum, and local-, regional-, and national-level nursing conferences. It is through these effective learning environments that students/mentees become socialized to becoming a researcher and learn how to develop the skills necessary to transform bedside nursing and continue to graduate school.[7]

Finally, the last way to mentor students is through the educator role. Through mentorship provided in this role, it is critical for students/mentees to learn theoretic foundations of teaching/learning, participate in teaching activities, attend faculty meetings as appropriate, and participate in service-related activities. Allow mentees to attend faculty meetings to learn the importance of shared governance and how decisions are made in academe, along with providing students with service-related opportunities, such as attending nursing information sessions and peer mentoring and tutoring in the learning center. These service opportunities are valuable not only to the student but also to the school because students are able to talk to potential students at open houses about their valuable experiences and provide a perspective that you cannot as a faculty member. In addition, by providing peer mentoring and tutoring in the learning center, students gain a theoretic background to the teaching/learning process during orientation but also valuable experience working with students individually and in groups in helping them grasp content in a variety of nursing, mathematics, and science courses. Finally, encourage mentees to attend educational Webinars, seminars, and conferences.

FUNDING

Funding not only entices students to join a research team but also serves to reward and value their critical contributions to the team. As a faculty member, try to obtain grant funding to pay at least 1 team member to work as an undergraduate research assistant. Although the pay may not be much, it does serve as an incentive for him or her to continue working with the team and provides them with experience similar to what he or she may be doing in graduate school. In addition, faculty should search for internal and external grants for their students. Not only does this provide a source of funding for mentees but also allows them to gain experience in grant writing. Grant funding can help fund mentee's attendance at conferences, along with their research projects.

DIFFICULTIES

Although mentoring nursing students is needed to develop the next generation of nursing leaders, it does not come without added work. For example, be prepared for mistakes to happen and for projects to take longer than you are used to. However, watching students transform into capable leaders is worth the wait. Although projects may take longer to complete and you need to spend valuable time coaching your mentees, you can see that the reward can be great because you are then a coauthor on a variety of peer-reviewed publications and presentations. In addition, you are preparing the next generation of leaders, while helping to prepare them for graduate school and to be your future colleagues.

Another area of difficulty is that mentees will often e-mail and come to see you with their concerns, whether professional or personal. Although you may not personally see this as an issue and may consider it a privilege to help mold students into future leaders, it is still important to set boundaries when needed and to clearly articulate your availability to them so you can accomplish other projects and responsibilities.

The next difficulty is that your mentees may want to conduct research on a variety of topics that you may not have expertise in. However, this is where you must use your resources and remember that even if you do not have content expertise, which you cannot have in every area, you may still be able to provide methodological support for the project, or at the very least lead them to resources to help them conduct the project. Although ideally, each mentee would work on projects related to your research interests, you must also let your mentees grow and turn into independent researchers in topics that interest them. Encourage "junior" members of your team to work on projects related to your interest area or areas, but after they complete a few of these projects with you, it is fine if they begin working on topics outside of your interest area. Encouraging this independence is critical as they develop into future leaders and prepare for graduate school.

The final difficulty that will be discussed is not to take on too many mentees. By taking on too many students, you will be providing a disservice to everyone on your team because they will not have your full attention and you will get frustrated trying to help everyone. Although you may not be able to help everyone, you can help match them with other mentors and resources and certainly check on them from time to time.

SUMMARY

For our nursing profession to continue to grow and strive in today's complex health care field, it is critical that we prepare students beyond the boundaries of the classroom and with cocurricular experiences to help them transform throughout the 5 Stages of Clinical Competence.[4] It is through these cocurricular experiences that nursing students get early socialization to the nursing profession in a variety of roles that they may not otherwise get exposed to during their schooling. Although mentoring undergraduate students may take more time and work than is *required* as a nurse faculty, the rewards are endless, ranging from objective measurements, including teaching support and publication of manuscripts. It also provides intrinsic rewards, because we use our privilege as nurse faculty to help prepare the next generation of leaders in our great profession.

REFERENCES

1. Graduatenursingedu.org. APRNs are making up for a shortage of doctors and RNs… while still being expected to fill their core role | how to become a nurse practitioner. [online]. 2019. Available at: https://www.graduatenursingedu.org/2018/08/aprns-are-making-up-for-a-shortage-of-doctors-and-rns-while-still-being-expected-to-fill-their-core-role/. Accessed May 28, 2019.
2. Kessler TA, Alverson EM. Mentoring undergraduate nursing students in research. Nurs Educ Perspect 2014;35(4):2.
3. APRNs are making up for a shortage of doctors and RNs… while still being expected to fill their core role. How to become a nurse practitioner. 2-264. Available at: https://www.graduatenursingedu.org/2018/08/aprns-are-making-up-for-a-shortage-of-doctors-and-rns-while-still-being-expected-to-fill-their-core-role/. Accessed July 30, 2019.
4. Tuomikoski A-M, Ruotsalainen H, Mikkonen K, et al. How mentoring education affects nurse mentors' competence in mentoring students during clinical practice–a quasi-experimental study. Scand J Caring Sci 2019. https://doi.org/10.1111/scs.12728.
5. Gazaway S, Gibson RW, Schumacher A, et al. Impact of mentoring relationships on nursing professional socialization. J Nurs Manag 2019;27:1182–9. Available at: https://doi-org.ezaccess.libraries.psu.edu/10.1111/jonm.12790.
6. Race TK, Skees J. Changing tides: improving outcomes through mentorship on all levels of nursing. Crit Care Nurs Q 2010;33(2):163–76.

7. Masters K, Gilmore M. Education and socialization to the professional nursing role. In: Masters K, Gilmore M, editors. Role devlopment in professional nursing practice. 4th edition. Burlington (MA): Jones & Bartlett Learning; 2017. p. 173–83.

8. Ousey K. Socialization of student nurses–the role of the mentor. Learning in Health and Social Care 2009;8(3):175–84.

9. Benner P. From novice to expert: excellence and power in clinical nursing practice. Hemel Hempstead (England): Prentice-Hall International; 2001.

APPENDIX 1: SENIOR NURSING STUDENT VIGNETTE

For almost 3 years, I have had the privilege of collaborating with Michael Evans, PhD, MSEd, RN, ACNS, CMSRN, CNE, the Assistant Chief Academic Officer and an Associate Teaching Professor of Nursing at Penn State University. Dr Evans has mentored me in multiple areas as a student nurse, such as nursing skills and socialization into the nursing profession, academic field, and research mentorship. The guidance Dr Evans has provided for me has been pivotal in my growth professionally, academically, and personally.

Dr Evans' guidance throughout my academic career path has been monumental in my progression as a student. Since the beginning of my college career, I knew I was interested in pursuing research in nursing. After I expressed my interest, Dr Evans has exposed me to multiple branches of research and scholarly activity. With his generosity, I have been able to pursue my dreams of scholarly endeavors by fully immersing myself in the realm of research and the potential it has to offer. Dr Evans has been an impetus and a role model because we collaborate as a team on literature reviews, case study publications, quantitative and qualitative research studies, grant writings, and poster formatting. His guidance has pushed me to pursue areas I would have never imagined to be possible as an undergraduate student. Dr Evans has also been an exemplary example by exhibiting the importance of presenting and displaying scholarly works through means of publications, presentations, and lectures. By mentoring me in these areas I was once foreign to, I have gained the knowledge and confidence to feel comfortable in engaging and participating throughout these experiences as an undergraduate student and years beyond after I graduate. Overall, this mentorship has taught me the importance of giving; 1 day I aspire to fulfill the same role as a mentor and provide endless opportunities and experiences to students like I have been fortunate enough to have been given.

APPENDIX 2: SOPHOMORE NURSING STUDENT VIGNETTE

Since the day I first met Dr Evans, he has taken it upon himself to take me under his wing as an advisor, mentor, and professor. He acts as my academic advisor and also as my mentor for the research team that he offered me to be a part of early on in my first semester at Penn State Scranton. Working with him has given me confidence to pursue my professional aspirations, pushed me to expand my knowledge, and given me opportunities to explore the nursing field earlier than most students get the opportunity to.

Watching the work Dr Evans does has given me the opportunity to witness the qualities that a good nurse, teacher, and mentor should have. Because of the influence he has had on me, I have become more confident as a student and future nurse. By being a part of this research team, I have learned valuable skills, such as how to search academic databases and find scholarly articles and how to collaborate on an academic manuscript. Although Dr Evans will let me know when something can be done better, he always offers guidance on how I can accomplish that, which pushes me to become a better student and researcher. Knowing that he will always help and encourage me gives me the confidence to research and experience things that may be out of my comfort zone, which will make me more well rounded in the future. I have also gotten the opportunity to be mentored by Dr Evans in a clinical setting. He works as a part-time nurse, and I shadow him every other weekend while he makes home health visits. I get the opportunity to practice introductory skills on the patients that he sees, and he offers guidance every step of the way. This makes me more confident to keep practicing the skills that I am learning and makes me certain that nursing is the right profession for me to pursue. By Dr Evans providing me this opportunity, I have gotten to learn and practice nursing skills that I would not have learned until the following year of my nursing education. To prepare for this experience, I leaned skills such as taking blood pressure, taking pulse and respiration rates, listening to heart and lung sounds, and taking pedal pulses. These are things that I would not have been able to learn until my sophomore year of college had Dr Evans not taken me under his wing and mentored me. I have been able to experience an aspect of the nursing field during my freshman year that allows me to get a glimpse of how everything works.

The relationship that I have built with Dr Evans through him mentoring me is one that I am extremely grateful for. He pushes me to be the best student, researcher, and future nurse that I can be, and he is always looking out for me whether I think he is or not. Because of Dr Evans taking me under his wing and mentoring me, I have been and will continue to be exposed to new information and countless opportunities that I otherwise would not have been able to experience.

APPENDIX 3: GRADUATE OR DOCTORAL STUDENT VIGNETTE

I have had the pleasure of working with Dr Michael Evans as a mentor during my undergraduate education as a nursing student, as a current PhD student, and as a novice nurse in my first position at a home health and hospice program. In each of these positions, mentorship has provided me with the opportunity to further my professional and clinical skills and experiences.

As an undergraduate student, I was introduced to my mentor via the campus honors program. In need of an honors project, I began working with Dr Michael Evans on his current research at the time, which was focused on self-symptom recognition in heart failure patients. Throughout my undergraduate education, I was given opportunities to attend local and regional conferences, conduct my own quantitative research study, publish periodicals, and perform numerous podium and poster presentations. Little did I know that this early exposure to nursing research via Dr Evans would carve out my path as an aspiring nurse researcher and lead me to pursue a PhD in nursing (something I had not previously known was an option). The experience from each of the academic activities from my undergraduate education under the mentorship of Dr Evans prepared me to enter the PhD program with an understating of the basics of research and knowledge dissemination.

Although I was fortunate to maintain a single mentor across multiple venues, other less formal mentors also provided assistance and insight into professional, academic, and clinical aspects of nursing. Each seasoned nurse or professor who acted kindly and offered guidance acted as an informal mentor and facilitated growth within the field. It is important for experienced nurses and those within leadership positions to understand their impact on students or novice nurses and how their actions can contribute to appropriate socialization and transition into more professional roles within nursing.

Sepsis Management in the Emergency Department

Sarah E. McVeigh, DNP, GCNS-BC, RN

KEYWORDS

- Sepsis • Sepsis management • Emergency department • Sepsis bundles

KEY POINTS

- Sepsis is a deadly and costly condition, but effectively managing sepsis in the emergency department (ED) can help to improve patient outcomes.
- A key part of sepsis management is improving compliance with sepsis bundles, which can be challenging in the ED setting. Bedside nurses in the ED have a unique opportunity to facilitate early identification and treatment of patients with sepsis, which are essential components to increasing sepsis bundle compliance and improving patient outcomes.
- Interventions reviewed in this article can help to decrease time to sepsis identification and treatments, along with standardizing care and ways to provide education and feedback.
- Nursing leadership also has an important role to help facilitate changes and removing barriers to sepsis bundle compliance.

Sepsis is one of the leading causes of death in hospitals.[1] Each year, more than 1.7 million Americans are diagnosed with sepsis and more than 270,000 people die from sepsis.[2] Sepsis is also the most expensive in-hospital condition treated, with a total spending of $23.7 billion dollars in the United States in 2013.[3] The Surviving Sepsis Campaign, established in 2002, created sepsis bundles for the treatment of sepsis with the overall goal of reducing the mortality rates associated with sepsis.[4] Sepsis bundle refers to a set of evidence-based practices for patients with sepsis and septic shock that when completed together help to improve the quality of care and outcomes.[4] Compliance with these sepsis bundles is associated with a 25% reduction in the risk of death and can reduce overall costs.[5–7] Improving sepsis bundle compliance requires a focused evaluation of different areas of sepsis management. Although improving sepsis management is an interdisciplinary effort, nurses at the bedside and in leadership positions play a vital role in early response, leading changes, and identifying barriers to sepsis bundle compliance (**Box 1**).

Compliance with sepsis bundles can be difficult due to the fact that sepsis is a complex and challenging condition to identify and treat. This is especially true in the emergency department (ED), where patients may present with symptoms that could

College of Nursing, University of Iowa, 50 Newton Road, Iowa City, IA 52242, USA
E-mail address: sarah-mcveigh@uiowa.edu

Nurs Clin N Am 55 (2020) 71–79
https://doi.org/10.1016/j.cnur.2019.10.009   **nursing.theclinics.com**
0029-6465/20/© 2019 Elsevier Inc. All rights reserved.

Box 1
Areas of sepsis management

- Early identification
- Early treatment
- Standardizing care
- Education
- Feedback

---

indicate many different diseases and conditions, often making an immediate sepsis diagnosis challenging. Despite these challenges, it is important to begin the treatment of sepsis as close to presentation as possible to improve outcomes for patients. For each hour that the completion of the sepsis bundle is delayed, the relative mortality risk increases by 4%.[8] Preventing this delay and improving outcomes for patients can be accomplished by making changes in 5 main areas of sepsis management. These areas include early identification, early treatment, standardizing care, education, and providing feedback. Overall improvement in sepsis management requires a multifaceted program that addresses each of these areas to ultimately improve patient outcomes.

EARLY IDENTIFICATION

Early identification and treatment is important for improving the outcomes of patients with sepsis.[4] This importance was recently highlighted by the recommendation from the Surviving Sepsis Campaign to initiate bundle elements within 1 hour of presentation (**Box 2**) compared with the previous goal of completing all bundle elements within 3 hours.[9] To help achieve this new goal, interventions are needed to improve early identification of patients with sepsis. The most common interventions are the use of an electronic sepsis screening tool, a computer-generated sepsis alert, and a nurse-driven triage assessment. Implementation of an automatic sepsis identification system within the electronic health record to screen for sepsis is a concept that has been shown to decrease the time it takes to identify that a patient has sepsis.[10,11]

Box 2
Surviving sepsis campaign hour-1 bundle

- Measure lactate (repeat if > 2 mmol/L)
- Obtain blood cultures before antibiotic administration
- Administer broad-spectrum antibiotics
- Initiate fluid resuscitation of 30 mL/kg for hypotension or lactate greater than or equal to 4 mmol/L
- Administer vasopressors if hypotensive during or after fluid resuscitation (maintain MAP $\geq$65 mm Hg)

Abbreviation: MAP, mean arterial pressure.

Courtesy of the Society of Critical Care Medicine, Prospect, IL and the European Society of Intensive Care Medicine, Bruxelles, Belgium.

The screening tool is built into the medical record to identify criteria for possible sepsis, and when a patient meets the criteria, it then creates an alert within the electronic health record. This allows for ongoing screening to occur during the patient's visit, and the use of this electronic sepsis alert has been shown to decrease the time until a patient is seen by a provider.[11] It is important for both provider and nurses to monitor for these alerts and to act promptly when alerts occur.

The use of a nurse-driven triage screening assessment is also something that has been shown to improve bundle compliance when used with an electronic sepsis screening alert.[10] The implementation of a sepsis screening in triage allows for earlier assessment of the possibility of sepsis based on vital signs and a suspected infection. This brief screening assessment can vary in specific questions, but often a positive screening requires 2 or more systemic inflammatory response syndrome criteria (**Box 3**) along with a suspected or known infection. This screening highlights the important role the triage nurse plays by helping to promote early identification. Use of the triage screening has been shown to help prioritize patients with sepsis and decrease time to antibiotic administration[12,13] (**Box 4**).

EARLY TREATMENT

Although early identification of patients with sepsis is critical, it is just as important to begin treatment as soon as possible. A barrier to this can be the high patient-to-nurse ratios in some EDs, dividing a nurse's attention and possibly delaying care.[14] The implementation of sepsis response teams is an option to provide additional resources and personnel to attend to the needs of a patient with sepsis in a timely manner. Sepsis response teams, which often include representation from medicine, nursing, and pharmacy, show variability in the process for activation, with some activating the response team based on the decision of the provider, whereas others allowing activation by the nurse.[15,16] Despite the variation in activation, the use of sepsis response teams as part of a multifaceted quality improvement project improved bundle compliance and reduction in mortality.[15,16] A similar concept of implementing a code sepsis is a way to quickly mobilize resources. One study showed a 27-minute decrease in time to antibiotic administration even though the code sepsis was not called until the patient was seen by a physician.[17]

Timely administration of antibiotics is an important aspect of early treatment. Delays in antibiotic administration have been associated with poorer outcomes in patients with sepsis.[18] Developing a process to improve the availability of antibiotics in the ED through the use of an automated medication cabinet has been shown to decrease the time until antibiotic administration and improve appropriate antibiotic selection.[19]

Box 3
Systemic inflammatory response syndrome criteria

Temperature greater than 38 C or less than 36 C

Heart rate greater than 90 beats per minute

Respirations greater than 20 per minute or $Paco_2$ less than 32 mm Hg

White blood cell count greater than 12,000 or less than 4000 or greater than 10% bands

Data from Bone RC, Balk RA, Cerra FB, et al. Definitions for Sepsis and Organ Failure and Guidelines for the Use of Innovative Therapies in Sepsis. *Chest.* 1992;101:1644-1655.

Box 4
Methods to improve early identification of sepsis

- Electronic sepsis screening tool
- Computer-generated sepsis alerts
- Nurse-driven triage screening assessment

A similar system, an automatic antibiotic dispensing system, was used in a different study that showed improved antibiotic availability and improved compliance with antibiotic administration.[20]

Nurse-driven protocols have also been used as a way to decrease the time until the start of treatment of patients with sepsis. Nurse-driven protocols allow bedside nurses to begin completing sepsis bundle elements when a patient meets specific criteria for possible sepsis. These protocols often include the completion of laboratory tests and blood cultures and can also include beginning fluid resuscitation.[10,11] Use of a nurse-driven treatment protocol has been associated with an increase in bundle compliance and specifically with a decrease in time to antibiotic administration.[17] A nurse-driven protocol has also been associated with a decrease in mortality.[11]

The process for a nurse-driven protocol varies in different studies. In one study, after a positive sepsis screening in triage, the triage registered nurse initiates laboratory draws and blood cultures and requests intravenous fluid orders if indicated.[10] This allows for timely completion of key sepsis bundle elements before evaluation by a provider. Other studies have the bedside nurse responsible for carrying beginning actions, such as laboratory work, before provider assessment[11,21] (**Box 5**).

STANDARDIZING CARE

Standardizing care is important to ensure that the care being provided aligns with the current evidence-based treatment guidelines found in sepsis bundles (**Box 6**). A common method of standardization is the use of order sets specific to sepsis that reflect the sepsis bundle requirements. The implementation and utilization of a standardized order set for patients with sepsis and septic shock is significantly associated with an increase in meeting the sepsis bundle requirements.[22] It is also important that nurse-driven protocols are also reflective of the current evidence-based treatment guidelines.

Use of a sepsis bundle checklist at the bedside is another method to help standardize care. The checklist serves as a tool for tracking the completion of sepsis bundle elements while providing a reminder of the required bundle elements and timeframes. In one study, a checklist was first the responsibility of the physician, but due to poor compliance with the checklist, the responsibility changed to a nurse-driven checklist.[23] Although no specific data on the use of a sepsis checklist by itself were found, it was included in several studies that showed significant increases in sepsis

---

Box 5
Methods to improve early treatment of sepsis

- Sepsis response teams/"Code Sepsis"
- Improved antibiotic standardization and availability
- Nurse-driven protocols

> **Box 6**
> **Standardizing care of patients with sepsis**
>
> - Evidence-based order sets
> - Sepsis checklist

bundle compliance and improved patient outcomes.[16,21,23,24] Nurses at the bedside can play a key role in helping to complete the checklist and ensuring that all sepsis bundle elements are being met in the correct timeframes. Use of the checklist can also help to communicate the care that is still needed during key times, such as during a patient handoff.

Examples of sepsis checklists can be found in published studies and through the Surviving Sepsis Campaign Website, with some key differences noted. One difference is although the Surviving Sepsis Campaign has moved to a recommended hour-1 bundle, Centers for Medicare and Medicaid Services (CMS) still requires hospitals to report on compliance with similar elements in longer time frames (**Table 1**). Another important difference between Surviving Sepsis Campaign and CMS is when to initiate the sepsis bundle checklist. The Surviving Sepsis Campaign recommends the use of the bundle for all patients with sepsis, whereas CMS requires bundle elements for patients with severe sepsis and septic shock.[9,25] This difference is further complicated by the new definitions of sepsis, based on the Sepsis-3 guidelines published by the Society of Critical Care Medicine in 2016, which no longer uses the term "severe sepsis."[26] Despite these differences in terminology and timeframes, the care elements in the bundles are the same with the exception of the focused reassessment by a provider in the CMS sepsis bundles.

EDUCATION

Providing education on sepsis and sepsis management is essential because of the complex nature of sepsis and also due to the changes of the definitions of sepsis and sepsis bundles. One method of education to providers and nursing staff is the use of formal educational sessions detailing the components and importance of sepsis bundles. Small group presentations, meetings, lectures, and other formats were used to help provide this education.[27,28] Other studies launched large educational campaigns focusing on both nurse and physician education on sepsis bundle components and timeframes.[11,17] The use of visual aids, such as pocket cards, brochures, and posters, were also used in these campaigns. ED nursing–specific training was observed in one

> **Table 1**
> **Centers for Medicare and Medicaid Services sepsis bundle requirements**
>
> | Within 3 h: | Within 6 h: |
> |---|---|
> | • Complete lactate level | • Repeat lactate level if lactate > 2 mmol/L |
> | • Complete blood cultures (before antibiotic administration) | • Administer vasopressors for persistent hypotension after fluid resuscitation |
> | • Administer broad-spectrum antibiotics | • Focused reassessment by provider after fluid resuscitation |
> | • Complete fluid resuscitation of 30 mL/kg for hypotension or lactate level $\geq$4 mmol/L | |

Data from Quality Net. SEP-1: Early Management Bundle, Severe Sepsis/Septic Shock Version 5.5. 2019. Available at: https://www.qualitynet.org/files/5d0d3986764be766b01038c7?filename=2_1_SEP_v5_5.pdf Accessed May 8, 2019.

study that focused on sepsis identification and standardized treatment protocols during simulations, as well as the use of critical language, empowerment to speak up, and escalation guidelines.[16] Although many studies shared varying educational interventions used to improve sepsis bundle compliance, little data are available to support the impact of specific educational interventions. This supports the use of a multifaceted education specific to the needs of the facility to improve bundle compliance.[14]

Education specific for nurses at the bedside should include training on helping to promote early identification and advocating for their patients. Nurses play a key role in advocating for their patients to help ensure that they are receiving correct and timely care. Training on how to verbally approach providers to ensure that they were aware of possible sepsis cases and the time goals for treatment was included as part of the nursing education in one study.[11] Education needs to also be provided to triage nurses to help ensure that proper sepsis screenings are being completed, especially concerning the component of identifying a possible or suspected infection. This determination can be based on a variety of factors and clinical findings on which nurses should receive education and training. The importance of these educational topics is highlighted through the results of one study that found that ED nurses often struggle to identify and escalate patients with sepsis, highlighting the need to provide nursing training specific to these areas.[29]

FEEDBACK

Communication of performance through feedback is a necessary tool for improving compliance with sepsis bundles. In the literature, there is variety in how this feedback is provided. One method of providing feedback is through reporting and posting information on compliance. Posting compliance data on an internal Website or dashboard was one method of providing feedback from studies with improved sepsis bundle compliance.[16,28] One study implemented providing feedback to nursing staff and to physicians through the posting of physician profiles related to their individual sepsis bundle compliance at staff meetings.[7]

Some studies articulated the implementation of direct feedback to the provider. Sending weekly text messages was one method used to provide feedback to providers regarding sepsis bundle compliance, emphasizing the specific bundle elements that had the lowest compliance. Sepsis bundle compliance increased from 12.7% to 53.7% during the period where weekly feedback occurred.[15] The use of scorecards or provider-based report cards was also identified as a method of direct provider feedback.[7,30] In one study, a scorecard was sent to the emergency room provider within 24 hours of the case, detailing the compliance with the bundle elements. Results from this study demonstrated an increase in bundle compliance from 43% to 64%.[30]

In the studies that provided feedback, the source of the feedback was often not specified and when it was, it was variable. One study used a physician champion to provide feedback to other providers and nursing staff, whereas the ED director sent letters of reinforcement, nonpunitive in nature, to providers who were noncompliant with the bundle elements. Another approach used a clinical nurse specialist for feedback to nurses and a physician leader for feedback to providers.[22] Although both of these studies showed increases in bundle compliance, there were no data specific to these varied feedback methods.

ROLE OF NURSES AS LEADERS

Hospitals have recognized the need to improve outcomes related to sepsis given high mortality rates and costs associated with patients with sepsis, but facilitating this need can be challenging. Although improving sepsis management is an interdisciplinary task, nursing is essential to lead changes to improve sepsis management. This is true for both nurses at the point of care and those in formal leadership positions.

Nurses at the bedside in the ED are an integral part of the multidisciplinary team that is needed to meet the sepsis bundle requirements. Beginning in triage, nurses will often have an opportunity to identify possible patients with sepsis and to advocate for these patients to be evaluated in a timely manner. Nurses need to be champions for improving sepsis management and work to initiate any protocols, such as nurse-driven treatment protocols and sepsis checklists, to help facilitate better outcomes for these patients. Nurses at the bedside can also be drivers to help initiate and support education to further knowledge related to sepsis management.

Nursing leadership also has a role in supporting and facilitating changes to improve sepsis management. One way is through an interdisciplinary sepsis taskforce to identify and implement changes. This taskforce should include representation from medicine, nursing, pharmacy, laboratory, education, infection control, and the quality department. Representation should also include members from both the ED and the inpatient side to help ensure a cohesive transition during the admission process to allow for completion of any remaining sepsis bundle elements and to help identify any potential barriers in that process.

Nursing leadership will also have a role in helping to address barriers that are identified while improving sepsis management. Possible barriers can include insufficient time and staffing due to the large amount of time and attention that is often needed to meet the bundle requirements. Another barrier is the understanding of current sepsis protocols, because both the definition of sepsis and sepsis bundle requirements have undergone changes in recent years. Lack of collaboration is also a barrier that is crucial to address because effective sepsis management requires interdisciplinary teamwork. Nursing leadership can anticipate these barriers and help to promote education, teamwork, and workflows to allow for improved sepsis management and bundle compliance.

SUMMARY

It is important to remember that improving sepsis management in the ED is a not a simple, one-step process. Sepsis is a complex condition to treat, and improving sepsis outcomes requires multiple improvement efforts in each area of sepsis management. Early identification and treatment are essential components to improving sepsis bundle compliance and patient outcomes and can be accomplished through using electronic sepsis screening tools and alerts, nursing-driven sepsis screening tools and treatment protocols, and sepsis response teams. Bedside nurses play a vital role in these areas and need to be included and used when improving sepsis management.

Although ensuring an early response to treatment is a priority, it is still essential that the standard of care is being met and that it reflects the evidence-based practices found in the sepsis bundle. This can be accomplished through use of standard order sets and sepsis checklists to help prompt reminders of these best practices. The use of education and feedback are also essential to facilitating improvements in sepsis management. Understanding the correct standard of care, the reasons for improvement, and promoting awareness of areas where compliance is not being met through the use of feedback can help to drive the changes needed to improve outcomes.

Nursing has a critical role in improving sepsis management in the ED. ED nurses at the bedside are able to help identify patients with possible sepsis early, promote timely evaluations of these patients, and help reduce time to treatment. Nursing leadership also has an important role in helping facilitate changes and removing barriers to improve sepsis bundle compliance. Working together as part of an interdisciplinary team, nursing can help drive the changes needed to improve sepsis management in the ED.

DISCLOSURE

The author has nothing to disclose.

REFERENCES

1. Liu V, Escobar GJ, Greene JD, et al. Hospital deaths in patients with sepsis from 2 independent cohorts. JAMA 2014;312:90–2.
2. Centers for Disease Control and Prevention. Sepsis: data and reports. 2019. Available at: https://www.cdc.gov/sepsis/datareports/index.html. Accessed May 1, 2019.
3. Torio C, Moore B. Healthcare Cost and Utilization Project (HCUP): statistical brief #204. 2016. Available at: https://www.hcup-us.ahrq.gov/reports/statbriefs/sb204-Most-Expensive-Hospital-Conditions.jsp. Accessed October 12, 2017.
4. Surviving Sepsis Campaign. About the surviving sepsis campaign. 2017. Available at: http://www.survivingsepsis.org/About-SSC/Pages/default.aspx. Accessed May 2, 2019.
5. Levy MM, Rhodes A, Phillips GS, et al. Surviving sepsis campaign: association between performance metrics and outcomes in a 7.5-year study. Crit Care Med 2015;43:3–12.
6. Noritomi DT, Ranzani OT, Monteiro MB, et al. Implementation of a multifaceted sepsis education program in an emerging country setting: clinical outcomes and cost-effectiveness in a long-term follow-up study. Intensive Care Med 2014;40:182–91.
7. Hoo WES, Muehlberg K, Ferraro RG, et al. Successes and lessons learned implementing the sepsis bundle. J Healthc Qual 2009;31:9–15.
8. Seymour CW, Gesten F, Prescott HC, et al. Time to treatment and mortality during mandated emergency care for sepsis. N Engl J Med 2017;376:2235–44.
9. Surviving Sepsis Campaign. Hour-1 bundle. 2018. Available at: http://www.survivingsepsis.org/Bundles/Pages/default.aspx. Accessed May 2, 2019.
10. Gatewood MO, Wemple M, Greco S, et al. A quality improvement project to improve early sepsis care in the emergency department. BMJ Qual Saf 2015;24:787–95.
11. McColl T, Gatien M, Calder L, et al. Implementation of an emergency department sepsis bundle and system redesign: a process improvement initiative. CJEM 2017;19:112–21.
12. Mitzkewich M. Sepsis screening in triage to decrease door-to-antibiotic time. J Emerg Nurs 2019;45:254–6.
13. Shah T, Sterk E, Rech MA. Emergency department sepsis screening tool decreases time to antibiotics in patients with sepsis. Am J Emerg Med 2018;36:1745–8.
14. Reich EN, Then KL, Rankin JA. Barriers to clinical practice guideline implementation for septic patients in the emergency department. J Emerg Nurs 2018;44:552–62.

15. Arabi YM, Al-Dorzi HM, Alamry A, et al. The impact of a multifaceted intervention including sepsis electronic alert system and sepsis response team on the outcomes of patients with sepsis and septic shock. Ann Intensive Care 2017;7:57.
16. Grek A, Booth S, Festic E, et al. Sepsis and shock response team: impact of a multidisciplinary approach to implementing surviving sepsis campaign guidelines and surviving the process. Am J Med Qual 2017;32:500–7.
17. Bruce HR, Maiden J, Fedullo PF, et al. Impact of nurse-initiated ED sepsis protocol on compliance with sepsis bundles, time to initial antibiotic administration, and in-hospital mortality. J Emerg Nurs 2015;41:130–7.
18. Seymour CW, Kahn JM, Martin-Gill C, et al. Delays from first medical contact to antibiotic administration for sepsis. Crit Care Med 2017;45:759–65.
19. Kalich BA, PharmD, Maguire JM, et al. Impact of an antibiotic-specific sepsis bundle on appropriate and timely antibiotic administration for severe sepsis in the emergency department. J Emerg Med 2016;50:79–88.e1.
20. Doerfler ME, D'Angelo J, Jacobsen D, et al. Methods for reducing sepsis mortality in emergency departments and inpatient units. Jt Comm J Qual Patient Saf 2015;41:205.
21. Moore WR, Vermuelen A, Taylor R, et al. Improving 3-hour sepsis bundled care outcomes: implementation of a nurse-driven sepsis protocol in the emergency department. J Emerg Nurs 2019;45(6):690–8.
22. Winterbottom F, Seoane L, Sundell E, et al. Improving sepsis outcomes for acutely ill adults using interdisciplinary order sets. Clin Nurse Spec 2011;25:180–5.
23. Nguyen HB, Lynch EL, Mou JA, et al. The utility of a quality improvement bundle in bridging the gap between research and standard care in the management of severe sepsis and septic shock in the emergency department. Acad Emerg Med 2007;14:1079–86.
24. Na S, Kuan WS, Mahadevan M, et al. Implementation of early goal-directed therapy and the surviving sepsis campaign resuscitation bundle in Asia. Int J Qual Health Care 2012;24:452–62.
25. Quality Net. Fact sheet SEP-1: early management bundle, severe sepsis/septic shock. 2016. Available at: https://www.qualitynet.org/dcs/ContentServer?c=Page&pagename=QnetPublic%2FPage%2FQnetTier3&cid=1228772869636. Accessed May 8, 2019.
26. Seymour CW, Liu VX, Iwashyna TJ, et al. Assessment of clinical criteria for sepsis: for the third international consensus definitions for sepsis and septic shock (Sepsis-3). JAMA 2016;315:762–74.
27. Kuan W, Mahadevan M, Tan J, et al. Feasibility of introduction and implementation of the surviving sepsis campaign bundle in a Singapore Emergency Department. Eur J Emerg Med 2013;20:344–9.
28. Whippy A, Skeath M, Crawford B, et al. Kaiser Permanente's performance improvement system, part 3: multisite improvements in care for patients with sepsis. Jt Comm J Qual Patient Saf 2011;37:483.
29. Harley A, Johnston ANB, Denny KJ, et al. Emergency nurses' knowledge and understanding of their role in recognizing and responding to patients with sepsis: a qualitative study. Int Emerg Nurs 2019;43:106–12.
30. Wozniak J, Lei Y, Dargin J. The effect of providing clinical performance feedback on compliance with sepsis bundles in the emergency department. Am J Emerg Med 2017;35:1772–3.

Using Geographic Information System Mapping in Emergency Management

Expanding the Role of Nurses in Home Based Primary Care

Judith R. Katzburg, PhD, MPH, RN[a],*, Sarah E. Bradley, MA[b],
Jason D. Lind, PhD, MPH[b], Jacqueline Fickel, PhD[c],
Diane Cowper Ripley, PhD[d], Michael K. Ong, MD, PhD[e,f,g],
Alicia A. Bergman, PhD[c], Marguerite Fleming, MPA[h],
Leon B. Lee, MA[i], Sarah A. Tubbesing, MD, MSc[f,j]

KEYWORDS

- Emergency management • Home-based primary care • Nursing • Veterans
- Vulnerable populations • Geographic information system (GIS)
- Implementation evaluation

Continued

[a] VA Health Services Research and Development, VA Greater Los Angeles Healthcare System, 16111 Plummer Street (10H3), Building 70, North Hills, CA 91343-2036, USA; [b] Rehabilitation Outcomes Research Section, James A. Haley Veterans' Hospital and Clinics, 8900 Grand Oak Circle (151R), Tampa, FL 33637-1022, USA; [c] VA Health Services Research and Development Center for the Study of Healthcare Innovation, Implementation and Policy, VA Greater Los Angeles Healthcare System, 16111 Plummer Street (152), Building 25, North Hills, CA 91343-2036, USA; [d] Veterans Rural Health Resource Center-Gainesville, VA Medical Center (151B), 1601 Southwest Archer Road, Gainesville, FL 32608, USA; [e] VA Health Services Research and Development Center for the Study of Healthcare Innovation, Implementation and Policy, VA Greater Los Angeles Healthcare System, 11301 Wilshire Boulevard, Building 500, Room 3213A, Los Angeles, CA 90073, USA; [f] Department of Medicine, David Geffen School of Medicine at UCLA, Los Angeles, CA, USA; [g] Department of Health Policy and Management, UCLA Fielding School of Public Health, Los Angeles, CA, USA; [h] Veterans Health Administration, VA Office of Reporting, Analytics, Performance, Improvement, and Deployment, 810 Vermont Ave NW, Washington DC 20420, USA; [i] VA Health Services Research and Development Center for the Study of Healthcare Innovation, Implementation and Policy, VA Greater Los Angeles Healthcare System, 11301 Wilshire Boulevard, Building 206, Room 219, Los Angeles, CA 90073, USA; [j] Home Based Primary Care Program, VA Greater Los Angeles Healthcare System, 11301 Wilshire Boulevard, Building 213, Los Angeles, CA 90073, USA
* Corresponding author.
E-mail addresses: Judith.Katzburg@va.gov; JKatzburg@gmail.com

Nurs Clin N Am 55 (2020) 81–95
https://doi.org/10.1016/j.cnur.2019.10.010
nursing.theclinics.com

Continued

KEY POINTS

- Veterans enrolled in the Veterans Health Administration (VHA) Home Based Primary Care (HBPC) program are a vulnerable population who may be at increased risk during emergencies.
- VHA-HBPC nurses, including frontline staff and managers, play a key role in emergency management of Veterans enrolled in the program.
- Geographic information system (GIS) mapping can be an important tool for patient management during the 4 phases of the disaster cycle: mitigation, preparedness, response, and recovery.
- The HBPC-GIS project is a quality improvement implementation and evaluation project that assesses GIS mapping for VHA-HBPC program management, including GIS mapping utility for emergency management.
- Preliminary results evaluating the innovative use of GIS mapping for emergency management by nurses at some VHA-HBPC sites indicate utility; further study is warranted.

INTRODUCTION

Nurse leaders can embrace innovations to advance patient care quality and safety. One technology garnering attention is geographic information system (GIS) mapping. Studies have examined the utility of GIS mapping for studying the epidemiology of disease and health care planning.[1–8] Nurses play an important role in emergency management,[9–14] but little is known regarding their use of GIS mapping for this purpose. This article presents GIS mapping as an innovation for emergency management by frontline nurses and nurse leaders to ensure the safety of Veterans enrolled in the Veterans Health Administration (VHA) Home Based Primary Care program (HBPC).

Veterans Health Administration Home Based Primary Care Program

The VHA-HBPC program was designed to serve Veterans with complex chronic conditions; this vulnerable population averages more than 8 conditions per patient.[15] VHA-HBPC consists of an interdisciplinary team of clinicians, generally including a physician, nurse practitioner or physician assistant, nurse, dietician, psychologist, social worker, occupational therapist, and pharmacist who provide ongoing primary care in the patients' homes.[15–17] Nurses function on the VHA-HBPC team as program directors, nurse managers, primary care providers, and case managers. Approximately 140 VHA-HBPC programs nationwide serve almost 38,000 Veterans (Davis D. National Program Director, VHA-HBPC program, personal communication, 2018).

The chronically ill and elderly are particularly vulnerable during emergencies, so disaster preparedness is especially important.[1,18–22] Patients who receive home-based care have high rates of chronic conditions, physical limitations, mental health issues, and electricity dependency to operate medical equipment.[15,23] In their varied roles on the VHA-HBPC team, nurses can play an important part in emergency management in all phases of the disaster cycle: mitigation, preparedness, response, and recovery (**Fig. 1**).[11,24,25] VHA-HBPC conducts emergency management at both the individual patient and organizational levels.

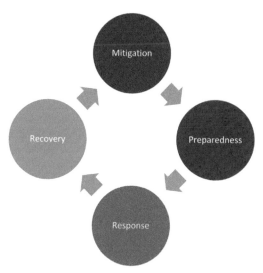

Fig. 1. The 4 phases of the disaster cycle.

The Disaster Cycle and Veterans Health Administration Home Based Primary Care: Mitigation and Preparedness

A national policy on disaster management has not been created for VHA-HBPC, although there are emergency management practice mandates.[17,26] The Joint Commission Environment of Care standard for emergency preparedness is seen as one driver for HBPC sites that are expected to develop emergency management plans. There is evidence that sites work together to develop plans.[17,26]

For the purposes of this article, mitigation is defined as risk prevention or reduction, including minimizing patient vulnerability to the effects of a disaster.[11,24,25] Preparedness is the totality of activities necessary to maximize emergency response capabilities at both the individual and the organization levels.[11,24,25] Aspects of mitigation and preparedness overlap, because emergency planning is part of both.

At the individual patient level, mitigation and preparedness efforts in HBPC can include nursing assessment of patient preparedness and assistance with a personal emergency preparedness plan (EPP).[11,24,25,27,28] The importance of having tools to assess patient preparedness and an EPP are noted in recent HBPC literature.[28,29] In assessing patient preparedness, VHA-HBPC team members, such as a primary care provider (PCP) or nurse case manager (NCM), consider the individual patient vulnerabilities and assign an acuity or risk score. Standardization of risk scores is recommended but has not been adopted across all VHA-HBPC sites.[27,30] PCPs or NCMs may also assist in the formulation of an EPP through their recommendations about necessary preparations and resources.[31] Outside services, including VHA-HBPC personnel, may not be available to the patient or family during or after an emergency.

At the organizational level, mitigation and preparedness are critical. Emergency management plans are a focal point of emergency preparedness at VHA-HBPC sites. Planning activities include identifying threats to the patient population using a hazard vulnerability assessment.[17] Environmental threats can pose variable dangers to patients given their diagnoses, acuity level, functional abilities, and whether they have a caregiver. After identifying threats and patient vulnerabilities, VHA-HBPC sites' plans use an all-hazards approach, which identifies all potential hazards and their impacts, to be prepared to respond to a variety of emergencies.[17,32] Plans must account for variability in staff capacity such as when environmental threats negatively affect staff census. Such shortages constrain VHA-HBPC leadership's ability to organize patient care.

The Disaster Cycle and Veterans Health Administration Home Based Primary Care: Response and Recovery

Response includes providing needed support to individuals and communities affected by emergencies.[24] Recovery is generally defined at the community level and entails helping communities to return to a functional level.[11,24,25] VHA-HBPC staff such as program directors, nurse managers, PCPs, NCMs, and social workers often coordinate patient evacuations and track patient locations. When conditions are again safe, VHA-HBPC staff resume home visits and assess patients' needs.

The Veterans Health Administration Home Based Primary Care Geographic Information System Mapping Project

GIS mapping is an important tool in emergency management and has been applied in a variety of health care settings, including for coordination of care and patient tracking during emergencies, to demonstrate the availability of community resources (eg, police and fire stations), and for general disaster planning.[1,7,33–37] These examples suggest the potential utility of GIS for emergency management in HBPC programs. The proactive use of available tools may lead to better outcomes during emergency events.[28]

The HBPC-GIS project is a quality improvement implementation and evaluation project that was created to optimize practice management through the provision of GIS software and training. The project mentors 30 HBPC programs in their use of Portal for ArcGIS, version 10.5, 2017 (Portal). The sites are diverse in rurality, HBPC team composition, and patient census. The HBPC-GIS project uses a multidisciplinary team to provide GIS training and technical support, which includes computer-based training modules and an online VHA forum for information exchange and downloading materials.

This article focuses on the role of nurses in emergency management at the 12 project sites where nurses participated in project evaluation. The 2018 project evaluation included questions about satisfaction with and use of GIS software, with specific attention given to use of GIS mapping for emergency management at their locations. The data from the participating nurses provide insight into GIS mapping utility and its application to emergency management for nurses working in VHA-HBPC.

METHODS

A mixed-method evaluation focusing on the feasibility, acceptability, and barriers and facilitators of HBPC-GIS mapmaking was conducted in the fall of 2018. The evaluation was designed to understand how HBPC staff created and used maps in HBPC practice management, and the potential impact on patient care activities. Given that VHA-HBPC staff interest in using GIS for emergency management was growing, the 2018 evaluation included this topic.

Quantitative data included a 27-item survey (Appendix 1), administered on RedCap, which was offered to all participating HBPC staff at the 30 sites. The survey consisted of 5 demographic items, 18 items related to general GIS implementation and satisfaction, and 4 items on using GIS maps for emergency planning. All nondemographic items were answered using a 5-point Likert scale: 1, poor; 2, fair; 3, good; 4, very good; and 5, excellent. Qualitative data included 24 semistructured telephone interviews with key HBPC program staff from each site. The interview guide (Appendix 2) focused primarily on activities related to emergency planning, including site goals, plans, implementation activities, personnel, contextual factors, mapmaking, map use, and barriers and facilitators to making and using GIS maps.

Analysis with a specific interest in nurse perspectives on GIS mapping in HBPC was conducted using data from the 12 sites where nurses either responded to the survey and/or participated in an interview. Results were compiled for nursing staff (in both frontline and leadership roles) from the 12 sites. Ten nurses from 9 of the 12 VHA-HBPC sites responded to the surveys. Thirteen nurses from the 12 VHA-HBPC sites participated in the interviews.

For survey results, descriptive statistics were calculated across the 9 sites, with continuous data presented as mean, standard deviation, and minimum and maximum values, and categorical data as frequency (percentage), using Microsoft Excel. Qualitative data analysis of the 12-site evaluation interviews was conducted by team members with expertise in qualitative analysis. Thematic categories were identified using a matrix analysis approach.[38] This approach involved categorizing and arranging data in an Excel spreadsheet and organizing them based on thematic categories, identified deductively using interview guide prompts, to produce case descriptions of each site. Consensus of thematic categories was achieved through discussion meetings with the evaluation team.

RESULTS
Survey Results: General Use of Portal for ArcGIS

Ten nurses (1 frontline staff nurse and 9 in management/leadership) from 9 HBPC-GIS sites anonymously completed the survey (**Table 1**). At the time of the survey, 80% (n = 8) of the nurses were using Portal to create maps, and 90% (n = 9) were using maps created with Portal for practice management or other HBPC activities. Most of the respondents (60%, n = 6) were using the software less than one hour per week. Respondents were asked to rate their experience with Portal from 1 (poor) to 5 (excellent). Satisfaction survey results are summarized in **Table 1**. Although nurses rated highly the ability to upload patient data to mapping software and the ability to create GIS maps (4.13; between very good and excellent), they were less enthusiastic regarding the user friendliness of the software (3.67; between good and very good). Training modules and training support were generally rated as good or better. Importantly, the nurses favorably rated the ability to use GIS maps for emergency preparedness (3.9; between good and very good) as well as the overall experience with GIS mapping use in HBPC (3.9; between good and very good).

Survey Results: Use of Portal for ArcGIS for Emergency Management

Survey questions assessed experiences using Portal for emergency management (**Table 2**). Nurse respondents indicated that, in 2018, 55% (n = 5) of their sites were using GIS mapping for emergency planning and 33% (n = 3) used GIS for emergency response. Nurses reported that sites were most commonly using Portal to prepare for flooding (33%, n = 3), severe winter storms (33%, n = 3), power outages (22%, n = 2), and excessive summer heat (22%, n = 2). At least 1 site had also used Portal to prepare for a wildfire, tornado, or earthquake. According to the nurses whose 3 sites used GIS for emergency

Table 1
Survey responses to questions regarding geographic information system use and training (10 nurses from 9 sites)

Topic	N	Mean Rating	SD	Range
Map Making				
Ability to upload patient data to mapping software	8	4.13	0.83	3–5
Ability to create GIS maps	8	4.13	0.83	3–5
Overall user friendliness of Portal for ArcGIS software	9	3.67	1.12	2–5
Using GIS Maps in Practice				
Overall ability to incorporate ArcGIS into HBPC practice	10	3.4	1.43	1–5
Ability to use GIS maps for program expansion	9	3.67	1.32	1–5
Ability to use GIS maps for boundaries and territories	10	3.90	1.1	2–5
Ability to use GIS maps in day-to-day travel plans	10	3.20	1.14	1–4
Ability to use GIS maps for emergency preparedness	9	3.89	1.05	2–5
Learning to Use Portal for ArcGIS				
Accessibility of training modules	9	3.78	1.09	2–5
Quality of training modules	8	3.50	1.07	2–5
Technical support	9	4.22	0.83	3–5
Monthly all-site calls	10	3.80	0.79	3–5
Facilitation calls with individual site	9	3.89	0.93	3–5
Pilot Project Participation				
Clarity of expectations	10	3.56	0.88	2–5
Ability of site to set goals for use of maps	8	3.25	1.16	2–5
Ability of site to achieve stated goals	8	3.38	1.3	2–5
Overall experience in 2018	10	3.90	0.88	3–5

Abbreviation: SD, standard deviation.
Likert scale with: (1) poor; (2) fair; (3) good; (4) very good; and (5) excellent.

response in 2018, they responded to 4 emergencies: severe winter storm (22%, n = 3), wildfire (11%, n = 1), flooding (11%, n = 1), and excessive summer heat (11%, n = 1).

Interview Results: Overview

Thirteen VHA-HBPC nurses participated in the qualitative interviews: 2 staff nurses, 1 NCM, 1 program coordinator, and 9 program directors. Nurses at 9 of the 12 HBPC-GIS project sites interviewed (75%) used Portal in some capacity for emergency management in the past 12 months. Nurses at the remaining 3 sites had all experimented with using Portal in emergency management, or had used it for emergency management in the past. HBPC-GIS sites are located in a variety of climates, with locations across the United States. Annual risk for particular emergencies varies by location. The most commonly mentioned emergencies across the 12 sites included flooding (83%, n = 10), winter snow and ice storms (75%, n = 9), and tornadoes (58%, n = 7). Power outages were also a common concern (50%, n = 6), especially for patients with conditions reliant on supplies such as oxygen or a ventilator or in cases of extreme temperature. Other emergencies discussed were varied and included wildfires, extreme heat, hurricanes, mudslides, and earthquakes. The nurses' experiences with Portal are presented within the framework of the disaster cycle phases, followed by participant-identified barriers and facilitators to GIS use for emergency management in VHA-HBPC.

Table 2
Sites using geographic information system mapping for emergency preparedness and response (N = 9)

Emergency	Sites (n) Using GIS for Emergency Preparedness	Percentage Using GIS for Emergency Preparedness	Sites (n) Using GIS for Emergency Response	Percentage Using GIS for Emergency Response
	N	%	N	%
Wildfire	1	11	1	11
Hurricane	0	0	0	0
Flooding	3	33	1	11
Power outages	2	22	0	0
Severe winter storm	3	33	2	22
Tornado	1	11	0	0
Earthquake	1	11	0	0
Tsunami	0	0	0	0
Excessive summer heat	2	22	1	11
Other	0	0	0	0
None	—	—	—	—

Interview Results: Mitigation and Preparedness at the Individual Level; Importance of Risk Assessment and Personal Preparedness Plan

Participating nurses had found several ways to use GIS as a tool to minimize patient vulnerability to potential disaster outcomes. Nurses at some HBPC-GIS sites described the importance of ensuring that patients and/or their caregivers have an EPP developed for how to handle an emergency when it occurs, including evacuation decision making. EPPs were commonly discussed with patients on admission and following an assessment of the patient's risk level. Some sites that have a regular hurricane or wildfire season would also revisit individual patient's EPPs on an annual basis in preparation for the increased emergency threat. GIS maps can be used to identify which patients are vulnerable to particular emergencies, such as those living in flood zones, so that patients can be provided with additional information about that threat, as was the case for a Southeastern site, where a nurse described, "When we know people live in bad flooding areas, when they live in a house that looks like it's going to blow over just, you know, in the average day's wind, we're planning already." Similarly, a staff nurse at a Southeastern HBPC-GIS location gave an example of using mapping ahead of tropical storms to know which patients are most threatened so that they can check in with those patients to make sure they have plenty of food, water, and medicine.

The importance of patients' and caregivers' awareness of needed supplies for sheltering in place was mentioned. HBPC staff provide patients and caregivers with relevant information and education about emergency threats, response, and available community resources before emergencies, and check in with patients following an emergency to ensure that supplies are adequate, including a backup generator if needed. Emphasizing the importance of nurses having a diversified toolkit for educating patients, a nurse from a Midwestern site said, "Registered nurses take the bulk of that responsibility on themselves because they're in the home more frequently than the rest. RNs [registered nurses] probably do 90 plus percent of the education in this area." GIS maps can be used to provide information about the location of community resources, including special needs shelters, and nurses showed the ability to use maps in this manner.

Interview Results: Mitigation and Preparedness at the Organizational Level; Identifying Threats, Map Use, and Staff Management

Interview respondents underscored the importance of emergency preparedness, with a focus on identifying common emergencies, providing a map that identifies patient location in relation to potential emergencies, and creating maps of community resources. One nurse, who serves as program director from a Southern HBPC-GIS site, explained: "[We are] not waiting until an actual emergency is declared before we do anything ... the proactive approach, it just makes tremendous sense to me in terms of anticipating problems ... These are, as you know, highly vulnerable people." Nurses expressed that GIS was one tool that they used in order to be proactive about emergency preparation and management in their VHA-HBPC programs. For example, mapping could be used to help identify which disasters were most common in the patient catchment area. Two sites, 1 in the Southeast and 1 in the Midwest, had begun to experiment with preidentifying other high-threat locations, such as common locations for lightning strikes; thermal hot spots; and forecasts for smoke, snowfall, and ice.

Nurses showed the ability to create maps containing extensive patient vulnerability information (eg, geographic location, diagnosis, acuity, functional capabilities, caregiver in the home, electricity dependence, risk score). By providing a visual representation of this information, GIS mapping enabled nurses' prioritization of high-risk patients for particular threats. Across sites, the most common high-risk criteria included dependence on electricity (eg, requiring a ventilator or refrigeration for medications) and lack of a caregiver in the home. For example, 1 Mid-Atlantic location had created maps both of their patients without caregivers (who must be contacted within 24–48 hours of an emergency event) and of patients reliant on oxygen (who will be at higher risk if power outages occur). A staff nurse at 1 Midwestern site explained,

> Right now, I could tell you how many Veterans, or where the Veterans sit, that are emergency category two and emergency category one ... when there's a disaster so we can reach them quicker, and if they're living in an area that is specifically going to be flooded or there's going to be a huge snow storm, maybe there's a blackout for whatever reason, we can look at that really quick on the map.

Using maps to identify high-risk patients enhances nurses' ability to direct their response efforts during an emergency. This ability made a significant difference for a New England site, where the program director (a nurse) expressed, "I found that in doing our drills that we didn't really need to waste time calling 300 patients, two-thirds who are probably 1 or 2 [low or moderate risk]. We really just needed to call those ones that are highest risk. So we really fine-tuned it down." Nurses who were not currently mapping their high-risk patients noted that they were interested in incorporating those types of maps in order to prioritize response during emergencies.

Several of the HBPC-GIS sites were using GIS mapping to provide a visual resource of community assets, such as police stations, fire stations, and hospitals. This resource included community locations intended to provide respite during emergencies, such as heating and cooling centers or special needs shelters. Nurses at sites that were not currently mapping community resources saw the value in producing maps of these locations.

Nurse managers can also use GIS maps to address emergency-related staffing challenges. For example, GIS maps can help in identifying nurses who will be affected by impending threats, to help plan for staff shortages and patient reassignments.

Interview Results: Response and Recovery; Importance of Geographic Information Systems

In addition to the utility of GIS for mitigation and preparation, participating nurses were able to use GIS for emergency response. One common use of GIS was the addition of live weather layers to track current weather events and their impact. For example, by accessing GIS data made available by the National Oceanic and Atmospheric Administration, nurses at HBPC-GIS sites could see in real time where in their patient catchment area a tornado had hit or could track the progress of a live event such as a hurricane or wildfire (**Fig. 2**). Importantly, especially for patients dependent on electricity, map layers could provide up-to-date information about where power outages are occurring. For example, a Midwestern program director reflected on a situation in which a patient had to be unexpectedly evacuated during a flood because of a loss of power. A staff nurse at a Southeastern program explained that, for them, "Where GIS mapping comes in really handy is in storms that don't affect the entire catchment." The nurse reported visually identifying which patients were affected based on real-time weather layers. A nurse at another Southeastern program was able to use an overlay of the trajectory of Hurricane Irma to follow

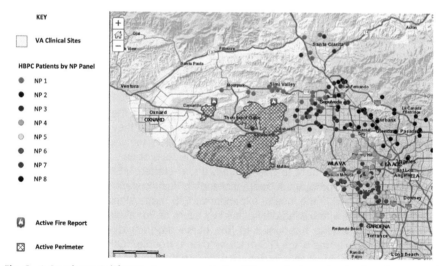

Fig. 2. A Southern California mapper created a GIS map to keep track of patients at risk from the Woolsey Fire of 2018. The Woolsey Fire started on November 8, 2018 burning more than 388 km^2 (96,000 acres) in areas of Los Angeles and Ventura Counties. Almost 300,000 people were evacuated. The Greater Los Angeles VHA-HBPC program created maps for nursing leadership and nurse practitioners (NPs) for the purposes of patient management given the fire threat as well as associated adverse effects such as poor air quality caused by smoke. (Map source: Portal for ArcGIS version 10.5 (2017), Environmental Systems Research Institute (Esri). Additional sources: HERE Technologies, National Geographic, United States Geological Survey, National Park Service, United States Geological Survey, Geospatial Multi-Agency Coordination.)

the path of the storm and associated flooding. Learning to use live layers to track weather was a popular future goal for nurses who were not already familiar with the technique.

Nurses did not discuss specific uses for GIS mapping during the recovery phase of emergency management. The most common use of mapping after emergencies was to review the response effort and identify areas for improvement. One program manager at a Southeastern HBPC-GIS site mentioned that they would like to use GIS mapping for coordinating future recovery efforts but they were not currently doing so.

Interview Results: Facilitators and Barriers to Use of Geographic Information Systems in Home Based Primary Care Emergency Management

When asked, most interviewed nurses indicated that they appreciated using GIS mapping in their emergency management. A program director at one Midwestern site enthusiastically expressed, "It's awesome. I think everyone should have it. I think it's an awesome tool and that it would benefit everybody." The mapping was seen to improve patient care by assisting communication with staff and leadership through a visual medium, and increasing program efficiency and decreasing response time during emergencies by prioritizing high-risk patients. However, a few sites saw value in using Portal for emergency management but were currently facing significant barriers. Three nurses indicated that although they saw the value of GIS mapping for other aspects of HBPC program management, they were not interested in using it in emergency management.

Although GIS mapping was being used at most of the participating nurses' VHA-HBPC sites, there were some common barriers to using GIS in emergency management. Barriers were primarily related to a lack of sufficient training in how to use the software, insufficient time to use the software, and technical issues. The amount of time required to learn GIS mapmaking skills was an important barrier. As one nurse/program director stated, "I'm still learning a lot about this … Every time I turn around, I'm learning something new about this map and how to make it work for me the best way possible."

Several sites agreed that the time required not only to learn the software but also to maintain their patient information in Portal was greater than they had originally anticipated. A New England program director experiencing limited staff time for Portal use expressed that, "I think the problem is that everybody is probably short-staffed and it's difficult to add another duty to overworked, under-staffed MSAs or PSAs [medical support assistants or program support assistants]." Issues were exacerbated by staff turnover that resulted in the loss of experienced GIS mapmakers. A Midwestern site expressed concern with having only a few key users of Portal when the staff mapper explained, "If something happened to [the nurse program director] or something happened to me, in terms of the GIS map, we'd be in trouble." Other sites encouraged their staff members to use the program, but the staff were not interested, as was the case for a Midwestern site where, "Their [staff] attitude was like, 'Oh, it's one more thing I have to do, one more thing I have to look at.'"

Several sites experienced technical difficulties with Portal that caused frustrations and limited overall usage. A New England site described its inability to properly incorporate a live layer of a snowstorm. A Southern site had recently lost all of its previously created maps in a server upgrade. The Portal is hosted online, which can cause issues during power outages. Staff at a Southeastern site found themselves creating hard-copy backups of information otherwise included on GIS maps because, "Post-storm it's highly dependent on having Internet access, whether or not you can get to your data in that format. So, if the power goes out or you lose Internet, you're dead in the water."

DISCUSSION
The Utility of Geographic Information System Mapping in Veterans Health Administration Home Based Primary Care

The results of the survey and interviews with nurses indicate that there are benefits of local-level GIS mapping in HBPC for emergency management. GIS was an effective tool in emergency management for both frontline nursing staff providing services to patients in their homes and nurse leaders serving as HBPC program directors or managers of HBPC nursing staff. Nurses used maps for individual patient emergency management, including helping patients prepare their personal emergency plans. Nurse leaders used maps to enhance emergency management of patient populations and/or staff.

At the patient level, using GIS for the creation of patient emergency or evacuation plans is not uncommon.[31,39] Nurses in this study made innovative use of GIS mapping to assist in proactive mitigation and planning activities, including assistance with patients' EPPs. Previous research has shown that home-based patients are not always prepared for emergency events, and community-dwelling elderly are at particular risk for low levels of preparedness for disaster.[26,40] Because of the increased vulnerability of this patient population, adequately preparing patients and their caregivers for emergencies is of utmost importance. Home-based care teams emphasize self-sufficiency during emergencies in partnership with the patients and/or their caregivers.[26] EPPs can bolster self-sufficiency. GIS mapping can assist in development of an EPP by identifying where community resources (including shelters) are located in advance. In addition, GIS mapping can benefit patients and caregivers by visually representing threats for particular emergencies, including flooding or an approaching storm.[41]

At the program level, proactive emergency management anticipates patient needs during a disaster event.[23] GIS enhanced proactive patient and staff management for these HBPCs. In an emergency event, there is often a limited amount of time to prepare for both patient safety and staff safety. Because nurses often act as leaders in disaster preparedness activities, home-based care nurses need to maximize their resources to enhance their effectiveness and efficiency in emergency response.[27] GIS can augment their efforts.

Project evaluation results indicate that nurses can use GIS to integrate individual patient information (eg, risk scores) with their locations in relationship to emergency and community resources, and/or proximity to the threat in order to prioritize patients for emergency management, including evacuation. The ability to visualize threats enables VHA-HBPC nurses to identify and prioritize patient and population vulnerabilities and plan accordingly. These maps also facilitate staff preparation and management for emergency response.

Satisfaction and Barriers to Use

The project evaluation results indicated that nurses were generally satisfied with the mapping experience. Some nurses were highly enthusiastic regarding the usefulness and importance of GIS mapping for emergency management in VHA-HBPC. Nurses who were not making or using the types of maps described earlier recognized their potential for future use.

Barriers to making or using maps were identified, especially the time-intensiveness of mapmaking, including tasks such as uploading patient-related data, mastering technical difficulties, and training challenges. A recent advance in mapping software at the VHA national level may ameliorate many of the reported barriers. The VHA Services Support Center has been working with a GIS analyst to develop an automated HBPC patient data report that has an integrated, user-friendly GIS mapping function. This automated report precludes the need for sites to upload patient data and simplifies map creation. Layers of environmental threats are included. This report is currently being pilot tested, and is anticipated to meet the needs of many HBPC-GIS users, including those who use maps to support emergency management.

LIMITATIONS

This project evaluation has limitations. Although triangulation of information from the survey and interviews bolsters results, it is not possible to draw generalizable conclusions because of the small number of implementation sites observed. The results may not accurately reflect the experience of nurses using Portal in VHA-HBPC nationally. These results cannot be extrapolated to all VHA-HBPC nurses, or to nurses working outside of VHA-HBPC.

SUMMARY

Although international standards exist, the United States currently lacks nationally adopted standards for disaster nursing practice and education.[42,43] In 2014, the Veterans Emergency Management Evaluation Center issued a call to action to improve the practice of disaster nursing, with support from the VHA Office of Emergency Management and the VA Office of Nursing Services. A dedicated group of volunteers have worked in the intervening years to advance disaster nursing, culminating in the establishment of the Society for the Advancement of Disaster Nursing (SADN).[14,44,45] There is ongoing research on the need for disaster nursing education and training in nursing schools, and throughout the nurses' careers, although GIS is rarely mentioned.[43,46] Further research on the efficacy of GIS as a tool for nurses, or more widespread development of automated reports providing GIS information, might eventually support inclusion of GIS in disaster nursing curricula.

Learning to use GIS mapping in VHA-HBPC for emergency management is a new and innovative concept. The HBPC-GIS project evaluation results suggest the utility of GIS for frontline nursing staff and nursing leadership in emergency management. The willingness to embrace innovation and learn new skills that would traditionally be seen as outside the scope of nursing is notable. However, additional research is warranted to further evaluate GIS use by nurses in HBPC and consideration of its application in home health and public health nursing.

ACKNOWLEDGMENTS

The HBPC-GIS Mapping Project was funded by the Veterans Administration Geriatrics and Extended Care Strategic & Transformational Initiatives. The authors are grateful to our colleagues who work in VHA-HBPC for their devotion and dedication to promoting the health of our Veterans enrolled in this program. The authors are thankful to Debra Wilson, RN, BSN, for sharing her technical expertise. The authors appreciate the efforts of the 30 VHA-HBPC sites participating in the mapping project. The authors wish to especially acknowledge VHA-HBPC nurses' efforts to ensure the safety of our Veterans during emergencies.

DISCLOSURE

This mapping project was funded by the Veterans Administration Geriatrics and Extended Care Strategic and Transformational Initiatives (V22.E16.691–4). The authors have no conflicts of interests to disclose. The contents of this article do not represent the views of the Department of Veterans Affairs or the United States government.

SUPPLEMENTARY DATA

Supplementary data to this article can be found online at https://doi.org/10.1016/j.cnur.2019.10.010.

REFERENCES

1. Aldrich N, Benson WF. Disaster preparedness and the chronic disease needs of vulnerable older adults. Prev Chronic Dis 2008;5(1):1–7.
2. Cowper Ripley DC, Kwong PL, Vogel WB, et al. How does geographic access affect in-hospital mortality for veterans with acute ischemic stroke? Med Care 2015;53(6):501–9.
3. Cowper Ripley DC, Litt ER, Jia H, et al. Using GIS to plan specialty health services for veterans: the example of acute stroke care. Journal of GIS 2014;6(3):177–84.
4. Cowper Ripley DC, Reker DM, Hayes J, et al. Geographic access to VHA rehabilitation for traumatic injured OEF/OIF veterans. Fed Pract 2009;28(10):28–39.
5. DeSalvo K, Lurie N, Finne K. Using medicare data to identify individuals who are electricity dependent to improve disaster preparedness and response. Am J Public Health 2014;104(7):1160–4.
6. Endacott R, Kamel Boulos MN, Manning BR. Geographic information systems for healthcare organizations: a primer for nursing professions. Comput Inform Nurs 2009;27(1):50–6.
7. Graves BA. Integrative literature review: a review of literature related to geographical information systems, healthcare access, and health outcomes. Perspect Health Inf Manag 2008;5:1–13.
8. Rodriguez RA, Hotchkiss JR, O'Hare AM. Geographic information systems and chronic kidney disease: racial disparities, rural residence and forecasting. J Nephrol 2013;26(1):3–15.
9. Baack S, Alfred D. Nurses' preparedness and perceived competence in managing disasters. J Nurs Scholarsh 2013;45(3):281–7.
10. Gowing JR, Walker KN, Elmer SL2, et al. Disaster preparedness among health professionals and support staff: what is effective? An integrative literature review. Prehosp Disaster Med 2017;32(3):321–8.
11. Hanes PF. Wildfire disasters and nursing. Nurs Clin North Am 2016;51(4):625–45.
12. Labrague LJ, Hammad K, Gloe DS, et al. Disaster preparedness among nurses: a systematic review of literature. Int Nurs Rev 2018;65(1):41–53.
13. Rowney R, Barton G. The role of public health nursing in emergency preparedness and response. Nurs Clin North Am 2005;40(3):499–509.
14. Veenema TG, Griffin A, Gable AR, et al. Nurses as leaders in disaster preparedness and response–A call to action. J Nurs Scholarsh 2016;48(2):187–200.
15. Beales JL, Edes T. Veteran's affairs home based primary care. Clin Geriatr Med 2009;25(1):149–54.

16. Edes T, Kinosian B, Vuckovic NH, et al. Better access, quality, and cost for clinically complex veterans with home-based primary care. J Am Geriatr Soc 2014; 62(10):1954–61.

17. Tubbesing S, Obal L, Brazier J, et al. Emergency preparedness for home based primary care senior veterans: lessons learned from previous experience. In: Cefalu CA, editor. Disaster preparedness for seniors. New York: Springer; 2014. p. 31–52.

18. Daugherty JD, Eiring H, Blake S, et al. Disaster preparedness in home health and personal-care agencies: are they ready? Gerontology 2012;58(4):322–30.

19. Dostal PJ. Vulnerability of urban homebound older adults in disasters: a survey of evacuation preparedness. Disaster Med Public Health Prep 2015;9(3):301–6.

20. Lamb KV, O'Brien C, Fenza PJ. Elders at risk during disasters. Home Healthc Nurse 2008;26(1):30–8.

21. Langan JC, Palmer JL. Listening to and learning from older adult hurricane Katrina survivors. Public Health Nurs 2012;29(2):126–35.

22. Phreaner D, Jacoby I, Dreier S, et al. Disaster preparedness of home health care agencies in San Diego County. J Emerg Med 1994;12(6):811–8.

23. Wyte-Lake T, Claver M, Dalton S, et al. Disaster planning for home health patients and providers: a literature review of best practices. Home Health Care Manag Pract 2015;27(4):247–55.

24. Jakeway CC, LaRosa G, Cary A, et al. The role of public health nurses in emergency preparedness and response: a position paper of the Association of State and Territorial Directors of Nursing. Public Health Nurs 2008;25(4):353–61.

25. Rose DA, Murthy S, Brooks J, et al. The Evolution of public health emergency management as a field of practice. Am J Public Health 2017;107(S2):S126–33.

26. Claver ML, Wyte-Lake T, Dobalian A. Disaster preparedness in home-based primary care: policy and training. Prehosp Disaster Med 2015;30(4):337–43.

27. Wyte-Lake T, Claver M, Dobalian A. Assessing patients' disaster preparedness in home-based primary care. Gerontology 2016;62(3):263–74.

28. Wyte -Lake T, Claver M, Tubbesing S, et al. Development of a Home health patient assessment tool for disaster planning. Gerontology 2019;7:1–9.

29. Wyte-Lake T, Claver M, Der-Martirosian C, et al. Developing a home-based primary care disaster preparedness toolkit. Disaster Med Public Health Prep 2016;11(1):56–63.

30. Zane R, Biddinger P. Home health patient assessment tools: preparing for emergency triage. Rockville (MD): Agency for Healthcare Research and Quality; 2011. Prepared by Abt Associates under Contract No. 290-02- 0600-011. AHRQ Publication No. 11-M020-EF.

31. Laditka SB, Laditka JN, Cornman CB, et al. Disaster preparedness for vulnerable persons receiving in-home, long-term care in South Carolina. Prehosp Disaster Med 2008;23(2):133–42.

32. Planning. Available at: Ready.gov https://www.ready.gov/planning. Accessed May 23, 2019.

33. Johnson R. GIS technology for disasters and emergency management. An ESRI white paper 2000. p. 1–12. Available at: https://www.esri.com/library/whitepapers/pdfs/disastermgmt.pdf. Accessed May 25, 2019.

34. Harrison JP, Harrison RA, Smith M. Role of information technology in disaster medical response. Health Care Manag (Frederick) 2008;27(4):307–13.

35. Bamford EJ, Taylor DS, Hugo GJ, et al. Accessibility to general practitioners in rural South Australia. A case study using geographic information system technology. Med J Aust 1999;171(11–12):614–6.

36. Litinger SH. Comparison of GIS-based public safety systems for emergency management. Presented at 24th Urban Data Management Symposium. Venice, Italy, October 27, 2004.
37. Lind JD, Fickel J, Cotner BA, et al. Implementing Geographic Information Systems (GIS) into VHA Home Based Primary Care. Geriatr Nurs, in press.
38. Miles MB, Huberman AM, Saldana J. Qualitative data analysis: a methods sourcebook. 3rd edition. Los Angeles (CA): Sage Publications; 2013.
39. Kirkpatrick DV, Bryan M. Hurricane emergency planning by home health providers serving the poor. J Health Care Poor Underserved 2007;18(2):299–314.
40. Gershon RR, Portacolone E, Nwankwo EM, et al. Psychosocial influences on disaster preparedness sin San Francisco recipients of home care. J Urban Health 2017;94(1):606–18.
41. Katzburg J, Wilson D, Fickel J, et al. Ensuring the Safety of Chronically Ill Veterans Enrolled in Home-Based Primary Care. Prev Chronic Dis 2019;16:1–4.
42. World Health Organization (WHO), Western Pacific Region, International Council of Nursing (ICN). ICN framework of disaster nursing competencies. Geneva (Switzerland): WHO and ICN; 2009. Available at. http://www.wpro.who.int/hrh/documents/icn_framework.pdf?ua=1. Accessed May 26, 2019.
43. Langan JC, Lavin R, Wolgast KA, et al. Education for developing and sustaining a health care workforce for disaster readiness. Nurs Adm Q 2017;41(2):118–27.
44. Langan JC, Lavin RP, Griffin AR, et al. From brainstorming to strategic plan: the framework for the society for the advancement of disaster nursing: a work in progress. Nurs Adm Q 2019;43(1):84–93.
45. Couig MP, Gable A, Griffin A, et al. Progress on a Call to action: nurses as leaders in disaster preparedness and response. Nurs Adm Q 2017;41(2):112–7.
46. Faruque F, Hewlett PO, Wyatt S. Geospatial information technology: an adjunct to service-based outreach and education. J Nurs Educ 2004;43(2):88–91.

Nurse Characteristics and the Effects on Quality

Lorraine Bock, DNP, FNP-C, ENP-C

KEYWORDS

- Emotional intelligence • Quality care • Nurse characteristics • Patient outcomes
- Staff nurse characteristics • Quality nursing care • Nursing outcomes
- Patient safety

KEY POINTS

- Quality of care and patient outcomes have been defined in many ways.
- Consistently the research has shown a correlation between nursing characteristics and quality care and patient outcomes.
- Factors not considered in this article include hospital teaching status, type of unit, unit skill mix, hospital safety culture, and total nursing hours per patient day.

INTRODUCTION

The delivery of quality care is a topic of conversation at every hospital, extended care facility, home health agency, and outpatient medical office across America. The conversation began in 1999 with the publication of *To Err is Human: Building a Safer Health System*.[1] In 2001, with the publication of *Crossing the Quality Chasm: A New Healthcare System for the 21st Century*,[2] the topic became front page news and work has continued with hundreds of experts studying the factors that enhance quality, shorten length of stay, reduce adverse events, and improve patient satisfaction scores. Nursing has been at the heart of most of this work because of the intimate relationship between patients and the nurses who care for them.[3]

With the focus on payment models and reimbursement requirements shifting from fee for service to the attainment of quality metrics, and financial penalties being levied for hospital-acquired complications, scrutiny on nursing care is increasing. It is widely accepted, particularly in the hospital setting, that nurses are the primary providers of health care and spend more time interacting with patients than any other health care team member. Nurses are being pressed to deliver higher-quality care, in hopes that it will shorten length of stay, avoid adverse events during hospitalizations, and reduce readmissions to maximize financial incentives for institutions and practices. When Medicare rolled out the Merit-based Incentive Payment System and Medicare Access and Children's Health Insurance Program Reauthorization Act (MACRA) programs and

College of Nursing, The Pennsylvania State University, 90 Hope Drive, Hershey, PA 17033, USA
E-mail address: lwm38@psu.edu

Nurs Clin N Am 55 (2020) 97–107
https://doi.org/10.1016/j.cnur.2019.10.007
nursing.theclinics.com

alternative payment models, such as the Quality Payment Program,[4] pressure increased on health care providers, nurses included, to deliver the most safe, timely, effective, efficient, equitable, and patient-centered (STEEEP) care[5] so preestablished quality metrics were achieved and reimbursement bonuses collected.

Characteristics of nurses delivering care at the bedside have been widely studied as a contributor to these factors. The research has confirmed that there are variances in patient outcomes when specific nursing characteristics are present or absent. Although most of the research has focused on the impact of demographic characteristics such as education level, specialty certification, and years of nursing experience on quality and patient outcomes, new research is emerging on the impact of job satisfaction, emotional intelligence, social skills, and personality characteristics. This article discusses both demographic and emotional characteristics of nurses and the impact that they have been shown to have on patient outcomes and quality of care.

Factors not considered in this article include hospital teaching status, type of unit, unit skill mix, hospital safety culture, and total nursing hours per patient day. It is notable that, in the studies reviewed, these factors were also mentioned as potential contributing factors to quality of care and patient outcomes, particularly total nursing hours. Multiple articles indicated that an increase in total nursing hours per patient per day decreased rates of falls and pressure ulcers.[6,7] The breadth of this article is limited to the impact of factors affecting nurses and nursing behavior.

DEMOGRAPHIC CHARACTERISTICS

Nurses play a critical role in the quality and safety outcomes of patients in hospitals.[6] Nursing workforce characteristics such as educational level, specialty certification, and years of experience have been investigated by researchers, with most studies finding a clear relationship between the variables and patient outcomes and satisfaction. Much of the data on nursing come from the National Database of Nursing Quality Indicators (NDNQI).[6]

Established by the American Nurses Association (ANA) in 1998, the NDNQI was developed to achieve 2 goals: (1) providing acute care hospitals with comparative information on nursing indicators that could be used in quality improvement projects, and (2) developing a database that could be used to examine the relationship between aspects of the nursing workforce and nursing-sensitive outcomes with data collected from more than 2000 hospitals in the last 21 years.[8] The hospitals report quarterly on nursing indicators, and an annual registered nurse (RN) survey supplementing these reports with additional information on nursing characteristics has been conducted since 2002 with more than 175,000 responses received.[8] The data from NDNQI is a self-selected sample because participation in the database is voluntary, but hospitals of all sizes and financial motivation from all 50 states and the District of Columbia contribute reports 4 times a year, making it widely representative of nurses in the United States.[6]

Nursing Experience

In Benner's[9] iconic book *From Novice to Expert*, she makes it clear that experience is essential for nurses to develop the clinical knowledge that is necessary for providing expert nursing care. Although the research is not in 100% agreement that experience results in better patient outcomes and performance, the research does support that inexperienced clinical nurses have more difficulty in recognizing patient complications and adverse patient event.[10] There has also been some disagreement on the exact point at which a nurse becomes expert, but a review of the literature showed that most researchers agree that a minimum of 5 years of clinical experience is required for a nurse to acquire the judgment and proficiency needed to be deemed an expert.[11–13]

Critical thinking ability and nursing judgment are bolstered by exposure to and repeated practice of clinical situations; however, the research is not definitive on the relationship between years of nursing experience and patient outcomes. O'Neill[10] notes in her dissertation that the rapid changes in technology add to the confusion. Falls, medication errors, the development of pressure ulcers, and 30-day mortalities were the most commonly studied nurse-sensitive outcomes in the studies reviewed for this article.

Despite the conventional wisdom expecting that patients being cared for by nurses with more experience will have improved outcomes compared with those being care for by the less experienced nurses, the research does not support this thinking. Aiken and colleagues'[14] research on mortality failed to show any effect on the length of time nurses were in practice or the 30-day mortality. However, the study did suggest that there were improved outcomes associated with nurses with Bachelor of Science in Nursing (BSN) degrees.[14] The book *Oncology: Breakthroughs in Research and Practice* also concluded that nurse experience could not be correlated either positively or negatively with patient mortalities in hospitals.[15]

When investigating medication errors, the research supports the belief that increased nursing experience reduces medication errors.[11,16] In the Blegen and colleagues[11] study, the results were definitive in showing that the higher the RN skill mix on a hospital unit, the lower the incidence of adverse events on that unit, specifically medication errors and patient falls. The reduction in error was up to 87.5%.[11] Another study revealed that nurses who had a previous experience with making a medication error were less likely to report an additional medication error than nurses who had never made a previous medication error.[17] Additional research is needed to determine whether this decrease in reporting is related to the negative repercussions that the occurrence of a medication error has on the nurse's career, or to some other factor.

When analyzing the impact of nursing experience on fall rates in hospitals and nursing homes, the relationship seems clear: more experienced nurses and nursing teams have fewer falls. In extended care facilities where the nursing staff had experience on the unit of greater than 1 year, the reduction in falls was statistically significant.[18,19] Other studies have also found significant relationships between more years of nurse experience and lower patient fall rates.[20] In the case of unassisted falls, falls that occur when there is no staff present to mitigate the impact of the fall on the patient or resident, research has also noted a decrease in the number of falls on units where nurses have more years of nursing experience. Another variable found to be associated with reduced falls is the tenure of staff on a specific nursing unit.[7,18] Although not a nursing-specific characteristic, it does bear mentioning that longer nurse tenure on a particular unit is likely reflective of a more experienced nurse.

Specialty Certification

Much of the work done to investigate the nursing characteristic of specialty certification and its impact on nursing-sensitive indicators has been done in the intensive care unit with nurses who are critical care certified. In 1976 the American Association of Critical Care Nurses (AACN) Certification Corporation launched the first specialty certification for nurses and there are now more than 110,000 certified acute and critical care nurses certified by the organization.[21] Another specialty certification whose impact on patient outcomes has been studied extensively is certified wound care nursing.

Florence Nightingale[22] wrote in 1859 that, if a patient developed a bedsore, it was a failure of nursing and not a consequence of the disease process. Pressure sore assessment is a widely accepted indicator of nursing quality of care. Multiple studies have shown a positive relationship between certified wound care nurses and the prevention and proper assessment of pressure ulcers.[23] Another study found that the prevalence of pressure ulcers decreased when nurses certified in wound therapy were present in a facility.[23,24] However, there was no significant relationship between certified and noncertified critical care nurses on skin breakdown.

Boltz and colleagues[25] found that, as the number of certified nurses on a unit increased, there was a reduction in the prevalence of falls. The study also found that the type of certification was irrelevant, with the exception of certification in gerontology, which did not translate into an impact on any of the nursing-sensitive quality factors measured. The study also did not support the reduction of other nurse-sensitive factors, including injurious falls, pressure ulcer prevalence, and restraint use with relationship to specialty certification rates on a unit.[25]

A limitation of these data may be that specialty-certified nurses had more continuing education and longer tenure as nurses,[26] which brings into question whether the specialty certification itself is the factor that improves outcomes, or whether it is the longer tenure and more continuing education that affects the results.

Educational Level

Nursing students eligible to take the National Council Licensure Examination are prepared in 3 different educational programs: associate degree, diploma, and baccalaureate. Nursing academia has suggested multiple initiatives to prepare nurses at only 1 educational level, the BSN, but there continues to be enrollment in associate degree or diploma programs. The question has long been whether the collegiate or hospital preparation of a nurse has an impact on patient outcomes and quality of care. The Institute of Medicine (IOM), now known as the National Academies of Science, made a recommendation in 2011 that hospitals should increase the number of BSN-prepared RNs after the publication of several studies that showed a clear correlation with RN preparation and improved patient outcomes. Aiken and colleagues[14] were able to show that, for every 10% increase in BSN nurses in staffing mixes, there was a resulting 5% decrease in mortality and failure to rescue.[26] However, there is a much smaller body of research that links BSN-prepared nurses to reduced medication error rates, reductions in pressure ulcer development, and lower infection rates.[10] Blegen and colleagues[27] were able to show that patients who were cared for by RNs prepared with a BSN had lower rates of pressure ulcers than those cared for by Associate's Degree in Nursing (ADN) or diploma-prepared RNs. The BSN nurses also had lower rates of failure to rescue than their non–BSN-prepared counterparts.

EMOTIONAL INTELLIGENCE, PERSONALITY CHARACTERISTICS, AND OCCUPATIONAL BURNOUT
Emotional Intelligence

Emotional intelligence, or the awareness that emotions drive behavior both positively and negatively and the importance of learning of how to manage those emotions, was first defined by Peter Salovey and John Mayer[28] and later immortalized by Dan Goleman[29] in 1996 in his book *Emotional Intelligence*. Emotional intelligence also requires a high level of self-awareness, self-management, empathy, and social skills.[30] Examples of employees with high emotional intelligence include nurses who are team players, positive and down to earth, focused, accountable, confident, and ego free.[31] In early nursing education programs, nurses were encouraged to conceal their emotions and it was considered unprofessional for nurses to cry with patients or show emotion of any sort.[32] It is now acceptable and even encouraged for nurses to show emotion in support of their patients and in the development of the nurse-patient relationship. Caring for patients has both physical and emotional responsibilities, and some literature suggests that nurses do not get adequate preparation to be able to provide appropriate psychological support for patients.[32] This inadequate preparation results in a lower level of emotional intelligence in some nurses.

Emotional intelligence training and education is not usually included in basic nursing programs, but experts agree that emotional intelligence evolves with experience and repeated interactions with patients.[33] Having good emotional intelligence helps nurses to maintain their own well-being and psychological health. It also helps nurses be better prepared and deal more effectively with their patient's needs. Nurses with high levels of emotional intelligence are more likely to show less emotional fatigue, have fewer psychosomatic symptoms, have better overall emotional health, and work better in collaborative teams.[33] However, some researchers have criticized the methods used in measuring emotional intelligence because of the variety of definitions. Criticism includes inconsistency in the definition of emotional intelligence, poor variability in the instruments used to determine emotional intelligence and those used to measure typical personality traits, and that most emotional intelligence assessment relies on self-reporting.[34]

There is a body of literature on the need for emotional intelligence in nursing leaders. In their literature review, Abraham and Scaria[35] were able to find evidence ranging from well-designed controlled trials to expert opinions that support the need for emotional intelligence in nursing leaders. Outcomes such as increased drive and passion, improved communication, less bullying on nursing units, and effective management of conflict are noted when nursing leaders show high levels of emotional intelligence. However, research on the impact of emotional intelligence on patient outcomes and quality of care is less prevalent.

Crowne and colleagues[36] pointed out that high levels of emotional intelligence in team members resulted in higher performance and improved team dynamics, which should translate to higher quality of care delivered to patients of the team, although no research could be found that documented this assumption. Wang and colleagues[37] were able to conclude that the higher nurses' emotional intelligence, the more likely the nurses were to avoid burnout and the longer they stayed in the workforce. This factor relates back to the characteristic of nursing experience and its impact on quality of care.

Personality Traits

There is a very small body of knowledge that discusses personality traits such as compassion, empathy, and calmness. Positive personality traits may have benefits for both nurses and patients.[32] It has been shown that nurses' decision making is affected by whether that nurse experiences compassion.[38] In 2001, Henderson[39] also suggested, in a study involving abused women, that the ability to be or not be emotionally involved with a patient may contribute to the quality of care that patient perceives. Most of the nurses in the study perceived that emotional engagement is a requirement of quality nursing care.

Self-awareness, a personality trait critical to the development of emotional intelligence, is mentioned repeatedly throughout the literature.[30,33,35] McQueen[32] brought attention to the need for nursing curriculums to include courses and exercises in self-awareness to develop this quality in students. Other personality traits mentioned in the literature that contribute to the quality of care delivered by nurses include motivation, compassion, coping strategy, the ability to collaborate with others,[33] authenticity, empathetic understanding,[40] and creativity.[36] Compassion is considered essential for nurses.[38,41] Von Dietze and Orb[38] attempt to define and quantify compassion by suggesting that compassion is not just a natural response to another person's suffering but a moral choice that requires mindful nurturing. The investigators go so far as to deem it an essential component of a person's core being in order to deliver professional care.[39]

Occupational Burnout

The quality of care delivered by a nurse with occupational burnout has been found to be lower than that of care delivered by nurses who are emotionally healthy and engaged in their jobs.[42] Problems documented in nurses with occupational burnout include, but are not limited to, low concentration, loss of hope, irritability, absence of energy, and emotional breakdown.[43] Loss of concentration leads to an increased risk of errors, including medication errors, missed opportunity to prevent falls, and inattention to schedules for patient repositioning resulting in an increased risk for pressure ulcer development. In a Japanese study that measured nurse burnout and then measured patients' satisfaction with their care, there seemed to be no correlation with the patients' perceived quality of care and the nurses' scores on the Maslach Burnout Inventory.[42] Nurses whose scores indicated they had occupational burnout received patient satisfaction scores similar to those of nurses who did not indicate on the assessment tool that they were experiencing occupational burnout.[42]

One study collected data from nurses in 6 countries: Germany, New Zealand, Canada, Scotland, England, Japan, and the United States.[44] The nurses were asked to rate their levels of burnout using a series of consistent survey instruments from Maslach and rate the quality of care they delivered on the last shift that they worked on another validated Maslach survey tool. The tools were all associated with the Maslach Burnout Inventory. Across all 6 countries, nurses who indicated high levels of burnout also perceived the quality of the care they delivered to be low[44] (**Box 1**).

IMPLICATIONS FOR NURSE LEADERS

Organizations have begun to consider the qualities of employees beyond the education and testing requirements when searching for quality staff. Employees who can maintain an "even-keeled" demeanor are sought after by many employers.[31] In a blog posted in 2017, Kathleen Pfeiffer,[45] a director for BAYADA Home Health Care listed the top 8 qualities she and BAYADA thought defined a great nurse, and included in the 8 were caring, empathy, self-awareness, and respect (**Box 2**).

Box 1
Nursing characteristics that positively affect patient outcomes

Tenure on the unit longer than 1 year

Nursing experience

Specialty certification

BSN preparation

Self-awareness

Emotional intelligence

Box 2
Eight qualities of a great nurse

Caring

Communication skills

Empathy

Attention to detail

Problem-solving skills

Respect

Self-awareness

Desire to keep learning

Data from Pfeiffer, K. 8 qualities of a great nurse. April 6, 2017. Available at: https://blog.bayada.com/work-life/8-qualities-of-a-great-nurse.

As the body of knowledge regarding the impact of personality traits and emotional intelligence on performance increases, organizations may incorporate ways to evaluate this during the interview process to assist in selecting the best candidates for open positions.[31] Given that evidence supports the belief that team dynamics have a significant impact on adverse outcomes on nursing units, the benefit of having employees who have high emotional intelligence and positive personality traits seems obvious. Nursing leaders responsible for hiring employees should develop interviewing skills that screen for emotional intelligence. Recruiterbox offers a list of 7 tips that can help interviewers identify employees who have high emotional intelligence[31] (**Box 3**).

The goal of achieving Magnet certification in hospitals is to create a supportive professional nursing care environment. Increasing the number of BSN nurses and requiring diploma and ADN RNs to attain their bachelor's degrees is common in hospitals seeking or maintaining Magnet status. Magnet hospitals use more BSN nurses; enjoy higher nurse satisfaction, presumably leading to less nurse burnout; and have better nurse retention then non-Magnet facilities. Since education level, low burnout scores, and longevity are associated with better patient outcomes, nursing leaders should be compelled to consider implementation of Magnet strategies even if the facility is not seeking the certification.

Box 3
Interviewing tips to screen for emotion intelligence

1. Make it part of the hiring process
2. Include it in job descriptions
3. Conduct group interviews
4. Let everyone give feedback
5. Ask insightful interview questions
6. Observe how a candidate behaves outside the interview room
7. Check references

Data from Anderson, D. Emotional intelligence: the most overlooked candidate skill. (2016). Available at: https://recruiterbox.com/blog/emotional-intelligence-overlooked-candidate-skill.

SUMMARY

For nearly 20 years, the quality of care being delivered to patients in hospitals has been under scrutiny. With nurses being the primary caregivers in these institutions, much of the research on how to improve quality has focused on the profession. Quality has been measured by a variety of methods, including fall rates, the development of pressure ulcers, medication errors, and the 30-day mortality. These measures are considered exclusively nurse sensitive. With increasing pressure on nurses to deliver higher-quality care with fewer resources, the characteristics of nurses and their impact on patient quality have been investigated by many researchers. Although most of the focus was on demographic characteristics such as nursing experience, certification status, and educational preparation, a new body of knowledge deals with emotional intelligence, personality characteristics, and occupational burnout.

The bulk of the research upholds the work done by Aiken and colleagues[14] and others, showing that educational preparation, the BSN degree as opposed to the associated degree or diploma preparation, affects quality of care. The researchers have been able to show that units staffed with a higher level of BSN-prepared nurses have higher quality scores as indicated by lower numbers of medication errors, fewer falls and pressure sores, and lower 30-day mortalities. None of the studies has been able to conclusively determine what factor in the BSN education makes this finding replicable.

Specialty certification also has an impact on the quality of nursing care delivered, but the research is not as consistent. Wound care certification and certification as a critical care nurse was shown consistently in studies to be a predictor of high quality of care. The more of any type of certified nurses on a unit translated to lower rates of patient falls in 1 study. However, the same study failed to show a reduction in other nurse-sensitive quality measures.

Nursing experience has also been shown to be a factor in the delivery of high-quality care when investigating nurse-sensitive quality measures. Although most of the studies failed to define the years of experience needed to be considered experienced nurse, they did show consistently that nurses with less experience have increased difficulty in recognizing impending deterioration in patients' condition and adverse patient events. Medication error rates have been showed to be lower in more experienced nurses; however, the finding that nurses who have reported 1 medication error in their careers are less likely to report a subsequent error may indicate that the data are unfairly skewed because of lack of reporting.

The work focusing on emotional intelligence, personality traits, and occupational burnout is in its infancy in nursing. Early findings have shown that high levels of emotional intelligence in nurse leaders lead to less occupational burnout and more job satisfaction. Although the data on emotional intelligence in bedside nurses are scant, it can be agreed that nurses who are not burned out and who are happy in the workplace deliver better care.

Personality traits are being investigated in conjunction with emotional intelligence. Compassion, empathy, self-awareness, and authenticity have all been identified in the literature as personality traits that have a significant effect on patients' perceptions of the quality of care they are receiving. Personality traits also have a significant impact on the ability of nurses to work in teams, and effective teams are a key component of the delivery of quality care.

In addition, nurse burnout has been studied as a predictor of quality of care. The early studies and findings show across the world that nurse burnout correlates negatively with the perception of high-quality care by nurses. However, the same study[44] showed that patients did not perceive a difference in the quality of care when their nurses scored high on the burnout inventory. It is clear that nurses are at the heart of the delivery of quality care in health care institutions. There are many factors that contribute to a nurse's ability to deliver care that is of high quality and results in high levels of patient satisfaction. More research is needed to further define the nurse characteristics that influence the outcomes of factors considered to be nurse-sensitive measures.

DISCLOSURE

The author has no conflicts to disclose.

REFERENCES

1. Institute of Medicine. To err is human: Building a safer healthcare system. Washington, DC: National Academies Press; 2019. Available at: https://www.google.com/search?source=hp&ei=W2JXXcLgE8OGsQWWu5ugBQ&q=to+err+is+human+iom&oq=to+err+is+&gs_l=psy-ab.1.0.35i39j0i67l2j0j0i67j0j0i67l2j0j0i20i263.5203.6438..7776...0.0..0.139.1420.0j11....2..0....1..gws-wiz.......0i131i67j0i131.P3RjNMnW4RA#spf=1566007905495. Accessed April 15, 2019.
2. Institute of Medicine. Crossing the quality chasm: a new health system for the 21st century. Washington, DC: National Academies Press; 2001. Available at: https://www.ncbi.nlm.nih.gov/pubmed/25057539. Accessed April 20, 2019.
3. Institute of Medicine. Keeping patients safe: transforming the work environment of nurses. Washington, DC: National Academies Press; 2004. Available at: https://www.ncbi.nlm.nih.gov/pubmed/25009849. Accessed May 3, 2019.
4. U.S. Department of Health and Human Services: Centers for Medicare and Medicaid Services. Quality Payment Program. Available at: https://qpp.cms.gov/about/qpp-Overview. Accessed April 15, 2019.
5. Polancich S, Poe T, Miltner R. Improvement interventions and the IOM aims for quality: STEEEP-7. Patient Safety and Quality Healthcare. Available at: https://www.psqh.com/analysis/improvement-interventions-and-the-iom-aims-for-quality-steep-7/. Accessed April 5, 2019.
6. Dunton N, Gajewski B, Klaus S, et al. The relationship of nursing workforce characteristics to patient outcomes. OJIN. 2007. Available at: http://ojin.nursingworld.org.MainMenuCategories/ANAMarketplace/ANAPeriodicals/OJIN/TableofContents/Volume122007/No3Sept07/NursingWorkforceCharacteristics.html?css=print. Accessed April 15, 2019.
7. Staggs S, Knight JE, Dunton N. Understanding unassisted falls: effects of nurse staffing level and nursing staff characteristics. J Nurs Care Qual 2012;27(5): 194–299.
8. National Database of Nursing Quality Indicators. Available at: www.nursingquality.org/. Accessed April 27, 2019.
9. Benner P. From novice to expert: excellence and power in clinical nursing practice. Menlo Park (CA): Addison-Wesley; 1984.
10. O'Neill MA. Relationship of nursing characteristics to quality outcomes [doctoral thesis]. Gainesville (FL): University of Florida; 2014.
11. Blegen M, Goode C, Reed L. Nurse staffing and patient outcomes. Nurs Res 1998;47(1):43–50.
12. Atencio BL, Cohen J, Gorenberg B. Nurse retention: Is it worth it? Nurs Econ 2003;21(6):262–99.

13. Burrit J, Stechel C. Supporting the learning curve for contemporary nursing practice. J Nurs Adm 2009;39(11):479–84.
14. Aiken LH, Clarke SP, Cheung RB, et al. Educational levels of hospital nurses and surgical patient mortality. JAMA 2013;290(12):1617–23.
15. Information Resources Management Association. Oncology Breakthroughs in research and practice. Hershey (PA): IGI Global; 2017.
16. Blegen M, Vaughn TE. A multisite study of nurse staffing and patient occurrences. Nurs Econ 1998;16(4):196–203.
17. Jember A, Hailu M, Messele A, et al. Proportion of medication error reporting and associated factors among nurses: a cross sectional study. BMC Nurs 2018. https://doi.org/10.1186/s12912-018-0280-4.
18. Shin JH. Nursing staff characteristics on resident outcomes in nursing homes. J Nurs Res 2019;27(1):1–9.
19. Lee SE, Vincent C, Dahinten S, et al. Effects of individual nurse and hospital characteristics on patient adverse events and quality of care: a multilevel analysis. J Nurs Scholarsh 2018;50(4):432–40.
20. Blegen M, Vaughn TE, Goode CJ. Nurse experience and education: effects on quality of care. J Nurs Adm 2017;31(1):33–9.
21. American Association of Critical Care Nurses. Available at: https://www.aacn.org/about-aacn. Accessed August 5, 2019.
22. Nightingale F. Notes on nursing. Philadelphia: Lippincott; 1859.
23. Bergquist-Beringer S, Gajewski S, Dunton N, et al. The reliability of the National Database of Nursing Quality indicators pressure ulcer indicator: A triangulation approach. J Nurs Care Qual 2011;1–10. https://doi.org/10.1097/NCQ.0b013e3182169452.
24. Hart S, Bergquist S, Gajewski B, et al. Reliability testing of the National Database of Nursing Quality Indicators pressure ulcer indicator. J Nurs Care Qual 2006; 21(3):256–65.
25. Boltz M, Capezuti E, Wagner L, et al. Patient safety in medical surgical units: Can nurse certification make a difference. Medsurg Nurs 2013;22(1):26–37.
26. Coleman EA, Coon SK, Lockhart K, et al. Effect of certification in oncology nursing nursing-sensitive outcomes. Clin J Oncol Nurs 2019;13(2):165–72.
27. Blegen M, Goode CJ, Park SH, et al. Baccalaureate education in nursing and patient outcomes. J Nurs Adm 2013;43(2):89–94.
28. Salovey P, Mayer JD. Emotional Intelligence. Imagination, Cognition and Personality 1990;9(3):185–211.
29. Goleman D. Emotional intelligence. Stuttgard (Germany): Holzbrinck Publishers, LLC; 1989.
30. Beydler KW. The role of emotional intelligence in perioperative nursing and leadership: Developing skills for improved performance. AORN J 2017;106:317–23.
31. Anderson D. Emotional intelligence: the most overlooked candidate skill. Available at: https://recruiterbox.com/blog/emotional-intelligence-overlooked-candidate-skill. Accessed August 5, 2019.
32. McQueen ACH. Emotional intelligence in nursing work. J Adv Nurs 2004;47(1):101–8.
33. Raghubir AE. Emotional intelligence in professional nursing practice: A concept review using Rodgers's evolutional analysis approach. Int J Nurs Sci 2018;5:126–30.
34. Carragher J, Gormely K. Leadership and emotional intelligence in nursing and midwifery education and practice: a discussion paper. J Adv Nurs 2017;73(1):85–96.

35. Abraham J, Scaria J. Emotional intelligence: the context for successful nursing leadership: A literature review. Nurse Care Open Acces J 2017;2(6):160–4.
36. Crowne KA, Young TM, Goldman B, et al. Leading nurses: Emotional intelligence and leadership development effectiveness. Leadersh Health Serv 2017;30(3): 217–32.
37. Wang L, Tao H, Bowers BJ, et al. When nurse emotional intelligence matters: How transformational leadership influences intent to stay. J Nurs Manag 2018;26: 358–65.
38. Von Dietze E, Orb A. Compassionate care: a moral dimension of nursing. Nurs Inq 2001;7(3):166–74. Available at: https://onlinelibrary.wiley.com/doi/abs/10. 1046/j.1440-1800.2000.00065.x. Accessed April 5, 2019.
39. Henderson A. Emotional labor and nursing: an under appreciated aspect of caring work. Nurs Inq 2001;8:130–8.
40. Freshwater D, Stickley T. The heart of the art: emotional intelligence in nursing education. Nurs Inq 2004;11(2):91–8.
41. Kelly LA, McHugh MD, Aiken LH. Nurse outcomes in magnet and non-magnet hospitals. J Nurs Adm 2011;41(10):428–33.
42. Chao M, Shih C, Hsu S. Nurse occupational burnout and patient rated quality of care: The boundary and conditions of emotional intelligence and demographic profiles. Jpn J Nurs Sci 2015;13:156–65.
43. Fischer SA. Developing nurses' transformational leadership skills. Nurs Stand 2017;31(51):54–6.
44. Poghosyan L, Clarke SP, Finlayson M, et al. Nurse burnout and quality of care: Cross-nationals investigation in six countries. Res Nurs Health 2011;33(4): 288–98.
45. Pfeiffer K. 8 qualities of a great nurse. Available at: https://blog.bayada.com/work-life/8-qualities-of-a-great-nurse. Accessed: August 5, 2019.

Sustaining the Development of Clinical Nurses Within a Magnet Organization

Mary Louise Kanaskie, PhD, RN-BC[a],*, Kristine A. Reynolds, MSN, RN[b]

KEYWORDS

- Staff engagement • Shared governance • Professional development
- Clinical nurses • Magnet organizations • Community engagement • EBP fellowship
- Reward and recognition

KEY POINTS

- Magnet-designated organizations enrich the development of clinical nurses through a commitment to shared governance principles.
- Engagement of clinical nurses in shared decision making promotes improved outcomes.
- Cultivating practice innovations and offering reward and recognition programs help to sustain clinical nurse development.

INTRODUCTION

The American Nurses Credentialing Center's Magnet Recognition Program provides the framework for the structure and processes that focus on the development of the clinical nurse in all aspects of nursing practice. The Magnet Recognition Program uses the term clinical nurse to describe those nurses who provide direct patient care.[1] The Magnet model provides the framework to guide institutions in achieving the following:

- Improving patient, family, and community outcomes
- Acting to ensure that clinical nurses are involved in every aspect of patient care decision making and removing barriers to improve practices and processes
- Creating and nurturing a structure that empowers nurses at all levels to be actively involved in developing standards of practice
- Involving clinical nurses in the development of practice models that are patient centered

[a] Office of Nursing Research and Innovation, Penn State Health Milton S. Hershey Medical Center, PO Box 850, Mail Code H101, 500 University Drive, Hershey, PA 17033, USA; [b] Penn State Health Milton S. Hershey Medical Center, PO Box 850, Mail Code H101, 500 University Drive, Hershey, PA 17033, USA
* Corresponding author.
E-mail address: mkanaskie@pennstatehealth.psu.edu

Nurs Clin N Am 55 (2020) 109–120
https://doi.org/10.1016/j.cnur.2019.10.008

- Creating a culture that supports evidence-based practice (EBP) and innovation[1]

Sustained commitment to the tenets of the Magnet model is the key to a successful nursing organization. Institutions that achieve Magnet designation are constantly attentive to maintaining the structure and resources to reach quality outcomes.

Accountability at all levels of nursing is visible in Magnet-designated organizations through actions that produce the best possible patient, organizational, and community outcomes.[1] Nurses accept accountability for clinical decisions when they are empowered to define their work and determine standards of care.[2] It is our belief that organizations who are most successful at developing clinical nurses are those whose leaders "walk the talk" on a daily basis. Nurse leaders support and cultivate the culture of self-governance.[3] As a result, clinical nurses engaged in shared governance activities, on unit and departmental councils, and also develop leadership knowledge and skills.[4] Nurse leaders who show the core values of shared or professional governance in all decision making are ensuring that the organization's culture will support clinical nurse engagement.

This article discusses the key elements of sustaining the development of clinical nurses through the experience of Penn State Health Milton S. Hershey Medical Center's Magnet redesignation journey. Narrative examples describe the development of clinical nurses through shared governance commitment, redesign of the Professional Practice Model, engagement and commitment of the registered nurse (RN) workforce through shared decision making, an EBP fellowship program for clinical nurses, cultivating practice innovations, addressing the health care needs of our communities, and recognition and reward programs. Key elements are shown in **Fig. 1**.

COMMITMENT TO SHARED GOVERNANCE

The role of shared governance in sustaining the development of clinical nurses cannot be underestimated. Shared governance is the foundation for excellence in patient care. When led by transformational leaders, shared governance empowers clinical nurses to take the lead on issues such as patient safety, clinical practice, professional development, education, performance improvement, and EBP.[2] Shared governance capitalizes on each nurse's knowledge of clinical practice and integrates the nurse's participation in decisions regarding practice standards.[5–7]

Nurses throughout the organization are important members in decision-making processes through involvement in organizational committees, councils, and task forces. The Department of Nursing through the Professional Practice Model and Nursing Care Delivery System has built the structure for organizational groups to have input and feedback from clinical nurses through shared governance. Clinical nurses, nursing leadership, and advanced practice nurses are invited to participate in organizational

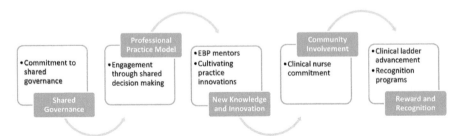

Fig. 1. Key elements for sustaining the development of clinical nurses.

and departmental committees, councils, and task forces based on their clinical focus, knowledge, and expertise or organizational role.

The nursing departmental council (Professional Nursing Practice Council) is facilitated by the Chief Nursing Officer and Magnet Program Director and has full authority for decision making within its areas of responsibility. This council has representatives from all inpatient units, ambulatory care, and interprofessional groups under the Department of Nursing. Representatives share information with their unit-based councils, which ensures the consistency of standards and provides a forum to address the unique needs of the patient populations served and the interests of clinical staff caring for them. The unit-based councils are chaired and cochaired by clinical nurses with the nurse manager acting as facilitator. The challenge for many institutions is finding a way to operationalize this concept and provide paid time for clinical nurses to be away from direct patient care to be involved in decision-making activities. The example presented in **Box 1** describes how to operationalize shared governance practices through organizational commitment.

PROFESSIONAL PRACTICE MODEL

Creating an environment for sustaining the development of clinical nurses begins with the advancement of a professional practice model (PPM) that resonates with staff at all levels. Success depends on the PPM being fully "embedded within the nursing culture and practices."[8]

Clinical nurses at Magnet-designated organizations are "involved in the development, implementation, and evaluation of the professional practice model."[1] Clinical nurses at our institution have practiced, collaborated, communicated, and developed professionally within the context of a PPM for more than a decade. In 2013, members of the Clinical Ladder committee were asked to review current literature on PPMs. The review of the evidence showed that the existing model had the required elements of a PPM but the model was complex and did not resonate with the clinical nurses. Further discussion led to consensus that simplification of the existing model was needed. A case example describing the redesign of the PPM by clinical nurses is presented in **Box 2**.

Description of the Professional Practice Model

The Nursing Care Delivery System (NCDS) is the central component of the PPM and embodies the nursing care and processes crucial to providing an extraordinary patient

---

Box 1
Case example: operationalizing the shared governance commitment

Clinical nurses from all inpatient units, procedural areas, and practice sites may serve as representatives on unit or departmental councils. These councils provide a formal mechanism for clinical nurses to effect positive and collaborative change throughout the organization. Opportunities are identified to improve the quality of patient care, efficiency of operations, and professional growth. Our shared governance model capitalizes on nursing knowledge and integrates participation in the decision-making process. Both unit and departmental councils provide members with an opportunity to meet on a regular basis.

Committee and council work hours are budgeted and scheduled to allow clinical nurse involvement within their full-time–equivalent positions. This time is tracked within the payroll system. The chief nursing officer and nursing leadership assist the organization in identifying which committees, councils, and task forces must have nursing representation to foster the multidisciplinary approach to work.

Box 2
Case example: redesign of the professional practice model

Clinical Nurse Involvement

Over several months, Clinical Ladder members worked on the PPM revisions. In addition, these clinical nurses worked with the Magnet Program Director to produce a video of the revised PPM. Clinical nurse participation in the PPM video production and content delivery shows integration of nursing practice with our mission, vision, and values. The video premiered at the Nursing Recognition Dinner that year. Nurses at all levels were assigned to view the video and complete the learning objectives on the learning management system.

Ongoing Evaluation and Implementation

The work of clinical nurses in evaluating and implementing the revised version of the PPM generated enthusiasm. Clinical nurses expressed having a better ability to communicate the integration of nursing practice into the delivery of quality care. The schematic is also used to communicate nursing care delivery at the unit level. The chief nursing officer and nurse managers use the schematic in a presentation to new employees that shows the connection to organizational strategic imperatives. These methods of using the PPM schematic are effective in introducing new employees to nursing practice, as well as keeping the importance of the PPM and NCDS at the medical center continually visible.

---

and family experience, depicted at the center of the schematic. Principles of the NCDS are stated in the wedges of the schematic (**Fig. 2**).

- Interprofessional collaboration indicates that clinicians function in teams and that effective communication is key to successful teamwork. Interprofessional collaboration results in positive outcomes for patients and families, and promotes a healthy work environment.
- Staffing and scheduling ensures that every patient is cared for by highly qualified nurses within a system of support that partners with all levels of nursing staff. Patient care assignments are made by matching knowledge and skill to fulfill patient care needs and promote continuity of care.

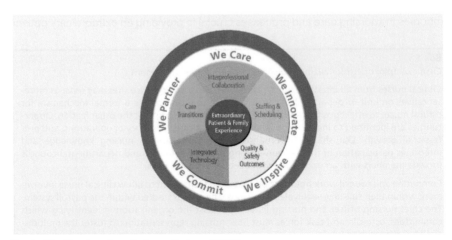

Fig. 2. The Nursing Care Delivery System (NCDS).

- Quality and safety outcomes result from the process and structure of the NCDS. Clinical nurses participate in quality improvement activities and apply evidence-based nursing care. Outcomes of nursing interventions are measured against national benchmarks.
- Integrated technology assists clinical nurses in providing patients with safe, quality care. In addition, the prudent use of advanced technology creates a better workplace for nurses and contributes to improvements in patient care.
- Care transitions focus on providing patients with the right care at the right time in the right setting. Clinical nurses and care coordinators assist patients and families along the care continuum to ensure holistic care that is part of the extraordinary patient and family experience.

In addition, the concepts and constructs of our nursing system are aligned with the Magnet model components: transformational leadership; structural empowerment; exemplary professional practice; and new knowledge, innovations, and improvements (**Fig. 3**).

The PPM schematic is visible to clinical nurses in their practice settings and introduced to new employees during orientation. Nurse leaders refer to the PPM in discussions with clinical nurses to show how the model provides a guide to meeting the organization's quality and patient safety goals and in providing an extraordinary patient experience.

Engagement and Commitment of Registered Nurse Workforce Through Shared Decision Making

Clinical nurses are important members in decision making at organizational, departmental, and unit levels. The participation of clinical nurses in these groups is vital to

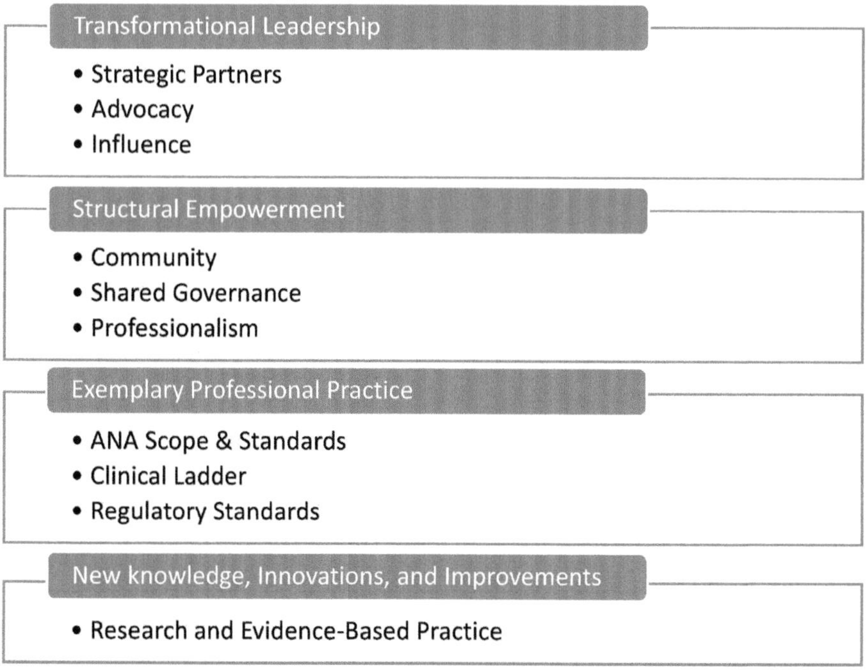

Transformational Leadership

- Strategic Partners
- Advocacy
- Influence

Structural Empowerment

- Community
- Shared Governance
- Professionalism

Exemplary Professional Practice

- ANA Scope & Standards
- Clinical Ladder
- Regulatory Standards

New knowledge, Innovations, and Improvements

- Research and Evidence-Based Practice

Fig. 3. Concepts and constructs of the NCDS aligned with Magnet model components.

the creation of a collaborative climate to standardize processes and to improve quality outcomes. Moreover, these groups are charged with creating a sustainable culture to improve patient safety and empower interprofessional teams to improve the patient experience.

An example of this collaborative culture was realized in the children's hospital. Recognizing that venipuncture is a primary source of anxiety for pediatric patients, an interprofessional team formed to standardize the experience with a therapeutic approach. A nurse and a physician with a passion to improve the pediatric patient experience developed the Lion's Pledge program to revolutionize pediatric venipuncture. **Box 3** describes the steps taken to develop the program and describes its outcome measures. Team members included perianesthesia clinical nurses, nursing vascular access team, child life specialist, and nurse educator and operational excellence staff. The Lion's Pledge interprofessional team was recognized as exemplary performance in the Magnet Recognition Program Summary Report[9] in September 2017 at the time of the third Magnet designation.

NEW KNOWLEDGE AND INNOVATION

"Magnet-recognized organizations use multiple strategies to create structures and processes that support a lifelong learning culture that includes professional collaboration and the promotion of role development, academic achievement, and career advancement."[1] Sustaining the development of clinical nurses includes providing opportunities for professional growth and participation in scholarly activities. Clinical nurses are uniquely positioned to identify innovative approaches to improve patient safety and nurse safety while improving patient outcomes. EBP mentors, quality improvement experts, and nurse scientists are important contributors to the scholarly advancement of clinical nurses.

Bringing Evidence to the Bedside

Providing clinical nurses with resources to find the best available evidence to answer their clinical questions about patient care interventions is an important strategy to promote best practices. The Advancing Research and Clinical Practice Through Close Collaboration model[10] purports that the development of EBP mentors is key to developing a culture that supports the integration of evidence into clinical decisional making. EBP fellowships are one method of developing EBP mentors within

---

Box 3
Case example: Lion's Pledge therapeutic approach to venipuncture in children

Clinical nurses assisted with the development of a care bundle consisting of 3 primary elements: pain management, comfort positioning, and distraction. Messaging focused on all elements, every patient, every time. Enculturation through the children's hospital included emergency department, phlebotomy, and radiology. To ensure sustainable culture change, Lion's Pledge was discussed monthly at shared governance councils and numerous interprofessional forums. A Lion's Guard of unit clinical nurses engaged as change agents was created to identify and remove barriers and share outcomes.

By using the care bundle as standard process, patient rating of discomfort during venipuncture decreased by 82%. Clinical nurses surveyed before and following Lion's Pledge implementation showed a 95% increase in agreement that the process is ideal and most therapeutic. Success rate of intravenous anesthesia induction increased by 72% and there was a 10% decreased in mask inductions.

organizations.[11,12] An immersion experience, conducted over 3 to 5 consecutive days, was the method used. The immersion consists of a structured curriculum and interaction with peers and mentors to learn important concepts about EBP and implementation strategies. The curriculum and outcomes are described in **Box 4**. The overall goal is to develop clinicians who use the best available evidence in making clinical decisions.[10] The fellowship concludes with instruction on dissemination of project findings through abstract writing and presentation development. EBP projects, research studies, and other scholarly projects are presented to internal audiences and at local, regional, and national conferences.

Cultivating Practice Innovations

Creating an organizational culture that encourages innovation in practice is another way of sustaining the development of clinical nurses. Clinical nurses are naturally innovative and, with sufficient resources, can develop patient care interventions that are effective, safe, and efficient.[13] "Innovation is the application of creativity or problem solving that results in a widely adopted strategy, product, or service that meets a need in a new and different way. Innovations are about improvement in quality, cost effectiveness, or efficiency."[13]

Innovation in practice is encouraged through recognition of nurses' unlimited capabilities and through allocating sufficient resources. The Innovation Award was developed in 2018 through a donation from the family of a former patient to be presented to a nurse or nurse-led team whose project best exemplify an innovation in patient safety or outcomes. The award criteria were modeled from the American Nurses Association (ANA) Innovation Award,[12] which is a monetary award intended "to provide one nurse or one nurse-led team with support to use translational research, development, prototyping, production, testing and implementation for an innovative product, program, project, or practice that is transformative to patient safety or outcomes."[14] An example of a funded innovation project is presented in **Box 5**.

CLINICAL NURSES' COMMITMENT TO COMMUNITY INVOLVEMENT

Penn State Health Hershey Medical Center complies with the Affordable Care Act and the requirements for Community Health Needs Assessment.[15] This requirement

---

Box 4
Case example: evidence-based practice fellowship for clinical nurses

Our institution's Office of Nursing Research and Innovation developed an EBP fellowship held over 3 consecutive days. The workshop provides the opportunity to "jump start" the EBP project. EBP fellows learn to search, analyze, and summarize evidence related to their practice question and develop an implementation plan for the practice change or improvement. Follow-up mentorship is done at planned intervals to provide ongoing support and additional information on project dissemination. Faculty for EBP fellowship includes nurses who are designated as EBP mentors, medical librarians, project management and quality improvement experts, and institutional data specialists.

Clinical nurses can apply to participate in the fellowship. The application process includes description of the clinical question of interest, brief description of the importance and relevance of the topic, and a letter of support from the nurse manager or direct supervisor. A recent group of EBP fellows represented inpatient adult acute care, critical care, and pediatric units. Projects included improvements in preventing device-related pressure ulcers, and several innovations, including the creation of an exercise program for hospitalized adults with cystic fibrosis and a protocol to reduce enteral nutrition interruptions for critical care patients.

Box 5
Case example: Innovation Award

The first recipient of the Innovation Award was a clinical nurse employed on the Neuroscience Critical Care Unit. Her project, "Creation of a Heat Map to Identify New and Existing Wellness Services for Stroke Patients," focuses on the initial data collection for the development of a mobile health application. The mobile health application seeks to link the gap between the discharge of a patient and follow-up appointment with effective, timely, and patient appropriate community wellness resources. The app will incentivize patients to achieve personal goals through their individualized plans of care.

---

extends beyond evaluation and assessment to include a hospital's strategy in using resources to build community engagement and to influence population health. Our regional community health strategy for 2019 to 2022 includes the following prioritized needs: extending the scope of behavioral health services, promoting healthy lifestyles, and disease management. As part of an academic medical center, our clinical nurses have the opportunity to partner with various departments in a variety of community outreach activities that address these community health priorities. A complete list of the community outreach programs is presented in **Box 6**.

Nutrition and Food Access Programs

A recent community member survey revealed that the client population we serve struggles with hunger and does not have a consistent source of sufficient and affordable food. Several initiatives have been designed to address some of this need: Food Box initiative, Community Garden, several regional food pantries, and farmer's markets. The Nursing Community Outreach Team saw an opportunity to incorporate healthy lifestyle messaging into the healthy foods offered at the farmer's market located on the grounds of the medical center. In addition, wellness-focus topics based on the Healthy People 2020 Leading Health Indicators[16,17] have been incorporated annually into the farmer's market. These topics are taught by unit-based teams of clinical nurses.

In collaboration with the Department of Health, the farmer's market combines agricultural, medical, and community resources focusing on healthy lifestyles related to childhood obesity, cardiovascular disease, stroke, women's health, and nutrition. The Nursing Community Outreach Team worked with the market director and health professionals in medicine, public health, and nutrition to establish a preventive health

---

Box 6
Clinical nurse commitment to community

Community outreach activities:
- Community and corporate health screenings
- School district department of education–required K–12 health assessments
- Pennsylvania State Farm Show (health screenings and education)
- Drive-thru flu vaccination
- National Drug Take Back Day
- Local and regional food bank partnerships
- Project homeless partnerships
- Food security programming
- No Texting campaign
- Bike Camp

---

booth at the market, combining healthy lifestyle coaching with nutritious market fare. Services include blood pressure measurements, body mass index screenings, and nutritional counseling with bilingual educational resources supplied. The farmer's market presents a unique opportunity to collaborate with on-campus entities as well as community partners toward addressing issues related to obesity and food insecurity by promoting access to healthy foods and nutrition education. Clinical nurses value this experience and enthusiastically participate. The farmer's market brings nurses together from the acute care hospital and ambulatory care sites with a shared goal.

RECOGNITION AND REWARD PROGRAMS
Clinical Ladder Advancement

Clinical recognition advancement programs are valuable methods for sustaining the development of clinical nurses and have been associated with improvements in nurse satisfaction and retention.[18] The Professional Clinical Ladder Program recognizes and rewards RNs for clinical excellence and provides a pathway for advancement of clinical nurses. Penn State Health's Milton S. Hershey Medical Center Professional Clinical Ladder Program is based on Patricia Benner's[19] explanation of clinical knowledge development. Benner[19] describes 5 levels of nursing practice based on clinical knowledge development. Recognizing that nursing is complex and difficult to describe solely by objective characteristics, narrative descriptions of practice in a particular situation are used to make visible the essence of nursing practice. All clinical nurses, following successful orientation and probationary period completion, are assigned to either level I (graduate nurse) or level II (competent nurse). Level III (proficient nurse) and level IV (expert nurse) are voluntary, initiated by the clinical nurse, and awarded additional monetary compensation. The professional clinical ladder program at our institution is in its third decade. The article "Clinical Ladder Program Evolution: Journey from Novice to Expert to Enhancing Outcomes"[20] describes the evolution through the first 20 years. Current revisions to the clinical ladder program are underway to recognize clinical nurses with advanced degrees who provide direct patient care.

Applications are reviewed by the Professional Clinical Ladder Committee led by clinical nurses who serve as chair and cochair and 1 nursing executive representative who serves as facilitator. The remainder of the committee is composed of clinical nurses, creating a true body of peers. Applicants develop a clinical portfolio showing level of practice and incorporating evidence from the following areas:

1. Independence and personal involvement that enhances professionalism
2. Accountability for competencies, areas of expertise, and levels of skill and knowledge
3. Subjective and objective data evaluation by the Clinical Ladder Committee
4. Impact of nursing interventions on patient outcomes

Applicants prepare 2 clinical narratives, which are a component of the portfolio. The narratives are reviewed to understand the nurse's level of knowledge development and clinical expertise. Criteria for each level are defined in domains of practice that reflect the ANA standards of professional practice.[21] In addition to the portfolio review, applicants participate in an in-person interview with clinical nurse peers who also serve on the committee. Clinical ladder level III and IV nurses are evaluated annually to ensure that their clinical performance is meeting standards of practice. The characteristic criteria of each level are added to the performance evaluation tool. Clinical nurses must maintain 90% of the characteristics of the practice level in order to be renewed at that level each year. Successful renewal of clinical ladder status is determined through a combination of self-appraisal, peer review, and management evaluation.

Recognition Programs

Meaningful recognition has been reported as a "significant predictor of decreased burn-out and increased compassion satisfaction."[22] Because meaningfulness is a subjective concept, the Department of Nursing makes a conscious effort to recognize those perceived differences. Recognition is given to all levels of nursing and their significant contributions are shared throughout the organization. The PPM described earlier supports the tenets for reward and recognition on many levels. The model recognizes clinical nurses for their contributions to the organization through teamwork and excellence, EBP, research, professionalism, and the clinical ladder. The Reward and Recognition Subcouncil ensures that nursing achievements are valued and recognized throughout the Department of Nursing and organization. The subcouncil's charter focuses on activities such as Nurses Week, the Nursing Recognition Dinner, spring and fall nursing awards, and recognition of unit-specific performance.

Annually, the Department of Nursing hosts the formal Nursing Recognition Dinner. This celebration is held at an elegant venue and is viewed by most clinical nurses as the event of the year. This event provides nurses the opportunity to network with colleagues and senior leadership to discuss the valued accomplishments achieved over the past year. Clinical nurses receive recognition in the following categories:

- Academic achievements
- Professional clinical ladder
- Professional nursing certification
- Professional and leadership activities
- Shared governance council leaders
- Publications and externally disseminated presentations

Box 7
Monetary awards and scholarships

Advanced Practice Clinician Excellence Award
  Recognizes advanced practice clinicians who show excellence in clinical practice and leadership in their roles.

Nursing Excellence Scholarship Award
  Supports professional career growth of nursing professionals currently enrolled or accepted in an accredited nursing program. Awards are given for each level: associate, bachelor, master, and doctoral degrees in nursing.

Award for Excellence in Nursing
  Supports nursing professionals who show a passion to continue their formal education in the pursuit of an advanced degree.

Oncology Nursing Excellence
  Supports the professional career growth of an adult oncology nursing professional.

Endowed Nursing Award
  Recognizes outstanding service and accomplishments of nursing staff.

Nursing Excellence Award
  Supports outstanding clinical nurses with awards to further their professional careers.

Nursing Community Service Award
  Recognizes outstanding commitment to community service by nursing employees.

- Distinguished internal and community awards
- Community service

The recognition dinner has grown with over 400 nurses invited annually and at least 200 nurses in attendance. In addition, awards are sponsored through the Development Office and presented during the Nursing Fall Awards Luncheon. The number of monetary awards presented annually varies based on endowments from community benefactors who recognize and acknowledge clinical nurses for the care they provide and their scholarly activities. **Box 7** presents a brief description of each monetary award.

SUMMARY

Development of clinical nurses through shared governance requires commitment of nurse executives and other organizational leaders. Commitment is shown every day in all activities of nursing departments and creates the culture that sustains professional governance. PPMs provide the description of the resources and relationships that enable clinical nurses to work collaboratively to provide quality care for patients, families, and communities. When clinical nurses participate in the design of the PPM, their engagement and commitment through shared decision making leads to quality outcomes and improvements in the patient experience.

Numerous clinical nurses who have served as council leaders in our institution later pursued advanced education in order to assume leadership roles. Some of these individuals have become clinical head nurses, nurse managers, or clinical practice nurse leaders. Others have chosen to remain at the point of direct care, where they serve as leaders in their practice specialties. Regardless of the path taken, clinical nurses' involvement in shared governance activities leads to increased awareness of leadership roles in nursing and builds confidence in their abilities.[4,23] The collaborative and team-building skills that are learned as council members and leaders will assist them in all future endeavors.

In addition, sustaining clinical nurse development is achieved through supporting EBP education for clinical nurses and providing professional resources to promote practice innovations and scholarly work. Reward and recognition programs that include professional advancement opportunities not only recognize competent and expert clinical practice but advance leadership development within the practice environment.

DISCLOSURE

The authors (M.L. Kanaskie and K.A. Reynolds) have no disclosures or funding to report and no commercial or financial conflicts of interest.

REFERENCES

1. American Nurses Credentialing Center. Magnet recognition program application manual. Silver Spring (MD): American Nurses Credentialing Center; 2019.
2. Porter-O'Grady T. Principles for sustaining shared/professional governance in nursing. J Nurse Manag 2019;50(1):36–41.
3. Moreno JV, Girard AS, Foad W. Realigning shared governance with Magnet® and the organization's operating system to achieve clinical excellence. J Nurs Adm 2018;48(3):160–7.
4. Lott T. Preparing clinical nurses for shared governance leadership roles. Nurse Leader 2016;14(6):403–8.

5. DiNapoli J, O'Flaherty D, Musil C, et al. The relationship of clinical nurses' perceptions of structural and psychological empowerment and engagement on their unit. J Nurs Adm 2016;46(2):95–100.
6. Joseph ML, Bogue RJ. A theory-based approach to nursing shared governance. Nurs Outlook 2016;64:339–51.
7. Kneflin N, O'Quinn L, Geigle G, et al. Direct care nurses on the shared governance journey towards positive patient outcomes. J Clin Nurs 2016;25:875–82.
8. Mensik JS, Martin DM, Johnson KL, et al. Embedding a professional practice model across a system. J Nurs Adm 2017;47(9):421–5.
9. American Nurses Credentialing Center. Magnet recognition Program® summary report. Hershey (PA): Penn State Health Milton S. Hershey Medical Center; 2017.
10. Melnyk B, Fineout-Overholt E, Giggleman M, et al. A test of the ARCC© model improves implementation of evidence-based practice, healthcare culture, and patient outcomes. Worldviews Evid Based Nurs 2017;14(1):5–9.
11. Mick J. Call to action. How to implement evidence-based nursing practice. Nursing 2017;47(4):36–43.
12. Fisher C, Cusak G, Cox K, et al. Developing competency to sustain evidence-based practice. J Nurs Adm 2016;46(11):581–5.
13. Kaya N, Turan N, Aydın GO. A concept analysis of innovation in nursing. Procedia-Social and Behavioral Sciences 2015;195:1674–8.
14. American Nurses Association (ANA). ANA Innovation Awards. Available at: https://www.nursingworld.org/practice-policy/innovation/ana-innovation-award/. Accessed May 17, 2019.
15. Centers for Disease Control and Prevention. Community health assessment and health improvement planning. Available at: https://www.cdc.gove/publichealthgateway/cha/index.html. Accessed May 31, 2019.
16. Centers for Disease Control and Prevention. National Center for Health Statistics. Healthy People 2020 Leading Health Indicators. Available at: https://www.cdc.gov/nchs/healthy_people/hp2020/hp2020_indicators.htm. Accessed May 29, 2019.
17. Building an appetite for health: nursing community partnership at local farmers market. Podium presentation. 2013 ANCC National Magnet Conference. Orlando (FL), October 3, 2013.
18. Warman G, Williams F, Herrero A, et al. The design and redesign of a clinical ladder program. J Nurses Prof Dev 2016;32(6):E1–9.
19. Benner P. From novice to expert. Am J Nurs 1982;82(3):402–7.
20. Burkett T, Felmlee M, Greider PJ, et al. Clinical ladder program evolution: journey from novice to expert to enhancing outcomes. J Contin Educ Nurs 2010;41(8):369–74.
21. American Nurses Association. Nursing: scope and standards of practice. 3rd edition. Silver Spring (MD): American Nurses Association; 2015.
22. Kelly LA. Effect of meaningful recognition on critical care nurses' compassion fatigue. Am J Crit Care 2017;26(6):438–44.
23. Fardellone C, Musil CM, Smith E, et al. Leadership behaviors of frontline staff nurses. J Contin Educ Nurs 2014;45(11):506–13.

Home Health Nursing Job Satisfaction and Retention

Meeting the Growing Need for Home Health Nurses

Delores (Dede) J. McCreary, DNP, RN, CNE

KEYWORDS

• Job satisfaction • Home health • Retention • Home health nurses

KEY POINTS

- The US Department of Labor predicts a 60.7% increase in the number of home health nurses needed by 2024.
- Turnover of nurses in home health has been increasing since 2000 and remains higher than average overall registered nurse turnover.
- Job satisfaction is the major determinant of retention.
- Patient relationships, autonomy and flexibility, and peer relationships are areas of high satisfaction for home health nurses.
- Workload and uncompensated time, documentation requirements, and salary are areas of low satisfaction for home health nurses.

INTRODUCTION

There is a growing need for home health care in the United States. The US Bureau of Labor Statistics projects that the compound annual rate of growth in employment for home health care from 2014 to 2024 will be nearly 5%, the highest for all industries.[1] The growth of home health will require a 48.6% increase in the number of registered nurses (RNs) employed in home health.[2] Home care agencies in all types and in all geographic regions are experiencing a shortage of nurses, with an increase in vacancies, difficulty recruiting, and turnover as high as 77%.[3] This turnover and difficulty recruiting is related to decreased job satisfaction for RNs in home care.[4] Since the year 2000, Medicare regulatory changes, which significantly increased documentation requirements and changed reimbursement from by-the-visit to a prospective predetermined amount, have contributed greatly to this decreased job satisfaction.[4] Since the

The Pennsylvania State University, 3000 Ivyside Park, 103H Sheetz Family Health Center, Altoona, PA 16601, USA
E-mail address: djm137@psu.edu

Nurs Clin N Am 55 (2020) 121–132
https://doi.org/10.1016/j.cnur.2019.11.002
0029-6465/20/© 2019 Elsevier Inc. All rights reserved.

implementation of prospective payment by Medicare in 2000, multiple nursing practice issues for home health nurses have been documented. Members of the National Association of Homecare as well as the Home Healthcare Nurses Association identified deep and serious concerns of home health nurses, such as excessive documentation and paperwork, including Outcome and Assessment Information Set (OASIS), isolation, need for professional development, and inadequate reimbursement.[5,6] These issues are making nurses think that they must focus more on documentation and reimbursement strategies than on patient care. Other concerns include the inability to meet patient needs within the number of visits authorized by payers, and productivity requirements necessitating 10-hour work days while only being paid for 8.[5] Home health and hospice turnover rates were the highest of all employer types included in a 2011 report by the Oregon Center for Nursing.[7] RN turnover rates in home health and hospice employers increased from 14.1% in 2004 to 24.6% in 2010.[7] In 2017, the national total RN turnover rate was 14.6%,[8] whereas the average turnover of home health nurses was 19.2%.[9]

The documented concerns of home health care nurses and the predicted growth in demand for home health care services requires leadership action. Decreased job satisfaction is a threat to the ability of home health agencies to provide nursing care.[4] Availability of home health care nursing services hinges on strategies used by nursing leaders to improve job satisfaction of home health care nurses.

REVIEW OF THE LITERATURE

Before the year 2000, home health nurses were highly satisfied with their work compared with acute care nurses.[10] However, this high level of satisfaction is waning. By 2004, home health nurses were among the most dissatisfied with their jobs.[11] This change in job satisfaction of home health nurses is attributed to significant changes in Centers for Medicare and Medicaid Services (CMS) regulations that have put demands on nurses in home health to complete excessive documentation and provide care within restrictive rules and regulations.[12–14] These changes have decreased job satisfaction and made it difficult for agencies to recruit and retain nurses.[3] With a significant increase in the demand for home health care predicted for the near future,[1] the need to retain home health nurses is essential. The major determinant of retention is job satisfaction.[15]

Factors Contributing to Job Satisfaction in Home Health Nurses

Studies relating to job satisfaction of home health care nurses are scarce and dated, but those that are published document a recurring theme of autonomy or independence, flexibility, and the relationship and time with the patients being the major satisfiers of home health nurses.[12,16,17] Of these 3 factors, autonomy is most consistently cited in the literature. In a convenience sample of 201 nurses in 19 home health care agencies, Tullai-McGuinness[4] found control over practice decisions and practice setting decisions accounted for 27% of nurse satisfaction. The category of autonomy and independence in Ellenbecker's Home Health Nurse Job Satisfaction (HHNJS) scale includes both flexibility and autonomy.[16] In a large study of 2459 nurses from a random sample of 123 certified home health care agencies in New England, the most frequently reported positive aspect of their job identified by participants was autonomy and independence.[16] The role that autonomy and independence plays in job satisfaction of home health nurses also emerged during earlier developing and testing of Ellenbecker's model of retention for home health care nurses.[13] In a qualitative descriptive study of 50 home care nurses with a mix of RNs and registered practical nurses in Ontario, "participants reported that having more authority over decisions related to client care contributed positively to their intent to remain (ITR)."[18] This study also identified the other 2 factors in the familiar triad: flexibility and relationships with the clients and families. A statewide survey of Oregon home health and hospice nurses conducted by the Oregon Nurses Association found that the primary sources of job satisfaction, identified by more than 85% of the nurses surveyed, were relationships with patient and families, professional autonomy and independence, and relationships with peers and coworkers.[19] In this study, 28% of the home health nurses said they were looking outside of their agencies for the same or similar positions. The impact of tightening regulation since 1999 may be affecting job satisfaction of home health nurses by decreasing autonomy and control over practice as agencies find the need to exert tighter control in order to meet requirements. "Nurses may not achieve autonomy if there are too many restrictive factors in the environment."[16] Sochalski[11] reported that home care nurses are among the most dissatisfied among all groups of nurses. "Interventions that may work to satisfy and retain hospital or institutionally based nurses may not be effective with home health nurses."[20]

Factors Contributing to Job Dissatisfaction in Home Health Nurses

Congruence is also found in the literature regarding the major factors contributing to dissatisfaction or the least satisfying aspects of being a home health nurse. These common factors are stress related to workload, excessive paperwork or documentation, and salary.[12,13,16,21] In a study of 340 nurses in 10 agencies, Ellenbecker and Byleckie[13] found that salary, benefits, stress, and workload were among the aspects that the nurses were the least satisfied with In addition to these, in a large, 3-year study of more than 2200 home health nurses that combined quantitative and qualitative data, Ellenbecker and colleagues[16] found multiple additional dissatisfiers, including poor relationships and communication with administration, car wear and tear, a lack of control, not feeling respected and valued, and poor communication with physicians and hospitals. Smith-Stoner and Markley[22] reported on a series of statewide conferences held to discuss home care outcomes with a special emphasis on strategies for retaining home care nurses. Their findings support Ellenbecker's[13] earlier findings regarding the importance of fair salary and streamlined, effective paperwork, but they do not identify these things specifically as areas of high dissatisfaction and they do not mention stress or workload.[22]

Examining a Home Health Agency

In order to address this issue, leaders at a Medicare-certified home health agency in central Pennsylvania pursued a quality improvement project designed to accurately measure job satisfaction of the nurses to address the increased turnover that the agency was experiencing. The method used a descriptive design to explore factors that contribute to job satisfaction of RNs in visiting staff positions in the home health department. Satisfaction levels of 8 components of job satisfaction were assessed using a standardized assessment survey instrument, the HHNJS scale. Narrative information was gathered by providing opportunity for comments on the instrument. The replies to these questions helped to clarify why individuals responded in a certain way and also provided opportunity to offer suggestions for improvement. Two additional open-ended questions were added to the end of the survey to collect information regarding what the RNs like the most about their jobs and what, if anything, may make them consider leaving. A demographic information section was developed and added to the HHNJS scale. The following items were included: employment status (full time, part time, or per diem), highest degree (diploma, associate's degree, bachelor's degree, graduate degree), number of years employed at the agency, and number of years of home health experience.

Methods

The HHNJS scale with added narrative prompts was used to gather information relating to the job satisfaction of home health nurses at this agency. The survey was developed into an electronic format and distributed to all home health staff RNs via e-mail. The e-mail explained the purpose and provided access to complete the survey. Completion of the survey was voluntary and anonymous. Qualtrics was used as the electronic platform for administration of the questionnaire. Completion of the questionnaire constituted consent. After completion of the survey, the data were analyzed and a report was prepared and presented to the agency leadership.

Instrument

The HHNJS scale was used for the quantitative data collection. The HHNJS scale was selected as the measurement tool because it is the only reliable and valid instrument available to specifically measure job satisfaction of home health nurses. It was developed and revised by Dr Carol Ellenbecker and colleagues[23] from 1998 to 2008. Multiple revisions have improved its psychometric properties. The latest version of the HHNJS was improved by adding, revising, and removing items along with reassignment of some items to subscales. This revision resulted in improved internal consistency and reliability with a Cronbach alpha value of .70, or greater, for all subscales with 1 exception (stress and workload) which was .69.[23] The HHNJS scale contains 8 subscales or constructs, 4 of which are relationship focused and 4 of which focus on other aspects of work.[23] The subscales correspond with the following 8 components of job satisfaction defined by Ellenbecker and Byleckie.[13]

Relationship with patients: a sense of connectedness, gratification, and accomplishment the nurse feels from working with patients.

Relationship with peers: the relationships nurses have with peers and the sense of social support, group communication, and perception of support they receive from peers. It is also conceptualized as social or group intimacy, social support, interaction or peer communication, and the perception of integration into the organization and the presence of a collegial environment.

Relationship with physicians: a sense of support in clinical decision making and positive interdependent relationship with physicians.

Relationship with organization: the relationships staff nurses have with the organization with supervisors and management.

Professional pride: a sense of pride and importance in the nurse's role inherent in the unique health care environment.

Autonomy and control: independence and control over hours of work, including scheduling, convenience, and flexibility; the amount of independence and discretion in conducting work. This component is also conceptualized as locus of control, individual responsibility, and task decision autonomy.

Stress and workload: the amount of pressure the nurse feels from the demands of work. Manageable demands make a job interesting and challenging; unmanageable demands that prevent nurses from meeting patients' needs create stress.

Salary and benefits: the monetary and nonmonetary compensation earned from work. Benefits include various types of insurance, leaves, and retirement funds. The degree of satisfaction includes an understanding of the possibility of salary and benefits elsewhere.[13(p779)]

The HHNJS scale consists of 30 Likert-type scale items that measure current levels of job satisfaction in the 8 components: relationship with patients, relationship with peers, professional pride, relationship with physician, relationship with organization, autonomy and control, stress and workload, and salary and benefits.[22] All items were rated on a 5-point Likert-type scale of 1, strongly disagree; 2, disagree; 3, neither agree nor disagree; 4, agree; and 5, strongly agree. Items with negative interpretation were reverse scored (5, strongly disagree).

Results

The survey was sent to 105 RNs and the response rate for the survey was 46.7%. Both quantitative and narrative survey results were analyzed. The mean overall job satisfaction score was 3.62 out of a possible high score of 5.00 (**Table 1**). Among the 8 components of job satisfaction, the 3 highest mean scores were for relationship with patients, relationship with peers, and autonomy and control (**Table 2**). The 3 lowest mean scores were for relationship with organization, stress and workload, and salary and benefits. Mean scores for the 3 questions relating to relationship with organization were 3.71, 3.65, and 2.8. The lowest score (M = 2.8, standard deviation [SD] = 1.05) was in response to the prompt, "I have the power to generate change in organizational policy at this agency." The remaining 2 components, professional pride (M = 3.83, SD = .93) and relationship with physician (M = 3.69, SD = .82) were in the midrange.

Narrative comments supported the quantitative findings. Of the comments categorized as facilitators (**Table 3**), themes with the highest percentage of comments were one-on-one patient care and patient relationship, peers, and flexibility. This finding corresponds with the highest quantitative scores being in the components of relationship with patients, relationship with peers, and autonomy and control.

Of the comments categorized as barriers (**Table 4**), themes with the highest percentage of comments were uncompensated time and documentation or computer system. These identified themes directly relate to the 2 lowest quantitative component scores: stress and workload and salary and benefits. Narrative comments related to salary were most often qualified with the number of hours worked. The theme of uncompensated time was seen as a barrier in the comments for 7 of the 8 components of job satisfaction. The only component for which this was not a barrier was relationship with physician. The theme of documentation or computer system was identified in the comments relating to 3 of the 8 components of job satisfaction. The remainder of themes were identified in only 1 or 2 of the 8 components.

Demographic information collected included years employed by the home health agency, years of experience as a home health nurse, job status, and level of education (**Table 5**). The number of years employed by the agency ranged from less than 1 to 11 to 20. Most (59%) nurses were employed by the agency for 3 years or less. The number of years as a home health nurse ranged from less than 1 to greater than 20. Nurses with 5 years or less of home health experience represented 53% of the sample, whereas 46% had 6 years or more of home health experience. Most respondents(80%) were full time. Nurses with an associate's degree were 43%, whereas

Table 1 Overall job satisfaction					
Component	n	Mean	Standard Deviation	Median	Mode
Overall	49	3.62	.85	3.72	3.68

Table 2
Job satisfaction components (high to low)

Component	n	Mean	Standard Deviation	Median	Mode
Relationship with patients	52	4.57	.51	4.80	4.80
Relationship with peers	51	4.29	.71	4.25	4.25
Autonomy and control	49	3.96	.97	4.00	4.00
Professional pride	49	3.83	.93	4.00	4.00
Relationship with physician	49	3.69	.815	4.00	4.00
Relationship with organization	49	3.39	.93	3.67	3.67
Stress and workload	49	2.63	.96	2.4	2.2
Salary and benefits	49	2.60	.98	2.6	2.5

those with a bachelor's degree were 41%. The mean level of overall job satisfaction based on demographic categories was analyzed and compared (see **Table 5**). No statistically significant differences were found for any demographic variable (**Table 6**).

Areas of Highest Job Satisfaction

Both quantitative and narrative project findings revealed that the components of job satisfaction that the nurses were most satisfied with were relationship with patients, relationship with peers, and autonomy and control. The theme of flexibility was the most frequently occurring narrative comment relating to the things nurses like the most about their job. Flexibility is included in the subcomponent autonomy and control in the HHNJS. These findings echo the recurring theme of autonomy or independence, flexibility, and the relationship and time with the patient seen in the literature as the areas of greatest satisfaction among home health nurses.[12,16,17] Satisfaction related

Table 3
Narrative themes: facilitators

Theme	Totals, n (%)
One-to-one patient care and patient relationship: being able to take care of 1 patient at a time and having an opportunity to get to know patients and establish a relationship with them	25 (24)
Peers: positive experiences and feelings related to peers	18 (17)
Flexibility: having some control over their schedule for the day, being able to make changes or flex their work hours	15 (14)
Like home health nursing or the agency: general expression of liking or enjoying home health nursing and/or the particular agency	14 (13)
Management or supervisor: positive comments regarding management or immediate supervisors	14 (15)
Physician relationship: being respected and valued by physicians	6 (6)
Autonomy and independence: being able to make independent decisions based on nursing knowledge and judgment	3 (3)
Support education: policies and processes mentioned that support further nursing education for nurses	2 (2)
Making a difference: having a positive impact on patients	2 (2)

Table 4
Narrative themes: barriers

Theme: Definition	Totals, n (%)
Uncompensated time: work time more than the 7.5-h day that salaried nurses are paid for or more than a reasonable visit time for nurses paid by the visit	62 (61)
Documentation or computer system: difficulties encountered related to the amount or difficulty of documentation requirements or the electronic documentation system	19 (19)
Benefits: aspects of the benefit package about which nurses express dissatisfaction	4 (4)
Opportunity for advancement: limited opportunities for advancement in the agency	3 (3)
Inability to effect change: not having a mechanism to contribute to make changes	3 (3)
Disrespect by physician: being undervalued or a nuisance to some physicians or their offices	3 (3)
Inequity of assignments: perceptions of patient load or assignments not being equitable among nurses	3 (3)
Restrictions on nursing judgment: stringent agency protocols or policies that do not allow for nursing judgment	2 (2)
Scheduling: difficulties encountered related to the scheduling processes	2 (2)

to peer relationships is also supported by previous studies. A statewide survey of Oregon home health and hospice nurses conducted by the Oregon Nurses Association found that the primary sources of job satisfaction, identified by more than 85% of the nurses surveyed, were relationships with patient and families, professional

Table 5
Demographics

	Category	n (%)	Mean Satisfaction
Years at Agency	<1	7 (14)	3.47
	1–3	22 (45)	3.40
	4–5	3 (6)	3.59
	6–10	9 (18)	3.59
	11–20	8 (16)	3.49
	>20	0	
Years as a home health nurse	<1	4 (8%)	3.48
	1–3	14 (29%)	3.38
	4–5	8 (16%)	3.40
	6–10	11 (22%)	3.57
	11–20	7 (14%)	3.43
	>20	5 (10%)	3.62
Job Status	Full time	39 (80%)	3.44
	Part time	2 (4%)	3.58
	Casual (as needed)	8 (16%)	3.61
Education	Associate	21 (43%)	3.45
	Diploma	5 (10%)	3.72
	Bachelor	20 (41%)	3.41
	Graduate	2 (4%)	3.68

Table 6
Comparison of demographic factors

Demographic Factor	Source of Variation	Sum of Squares	df	Mean Square	F	Sig
Years at agency	Between groups	.300	4	.075	.720	.583
	Within groups	4.586	44	.104	—	—
	Total	4.887	48	—	—	—
Years as a home health nurse	Between groups	.387	5	.077	.739	.598
	Within groups	4.500	43	.105	—	—
	Total	4.887	48	—	—	—
Job status	Between groups	.224	2	.112	1.106	.340
	Within groups	4.662	46	.101	—	—
	Total	4.887	48	—	—	—
Education level	Between groups	.479	3	.160	1.596	.204
	Within groups	4.405	44	.100	—	—
	Total	4.884	47	—	—	—

Abbreviation: df, degrees of freedom.

autonomy and independence, and relationships with peers and coworkers.[19] The fact that the level of nurse satisfaction related to the subcomponent autonomy and control was the lowest of the top 3 satisfaction scores may reflect the tight controls. "Nurses may not achieve autonomy if there are too many restrictive factors in the environment."[16] It is significant to note that, despite the high level of positive comments or facilitators related to peer and patient relationships, negative comments or barriers also co-occurred. These negative comments and barriers related to the theme of uncompensated time caused by high patient load that interferes with patient and peer relationships, a theme that was echoed in other areas in the survey.

Areas of Lowest Job Satisfaction

The components of job satisfaction with which the respondents were least satisfied were, in descending order, relationship with organization, stress and workload, and salary and benefits. These findings are also supported by the literature. Major factors contributing to dissatisfaction or the least satisfying aspects of being a home health nurse are stress related to workload, excessive paperwork or documentation, and salary.[12,13,16,21]

Relationship with organization was in the bottom 3 components of satisfaction, with an overall mean score of 3.39. Analysis of the 3 individual prompts measuring this component reveals that the lowest scoring prompt was, "I have the power to generate change in organizational policy at this agency," with the mean score of 2.8. This individual item mean is much lower than the means for the other 2 items for this domain, which were 3.71 and 3.65. This finding reveals a specific area of dissatisfaction for which improvement can have a significant impact on satisfaction and retention of nurses. Ellenbecker and Cushman[21] found that no intervention studied affected intent to stay but that shared decision making was the only intervention to have a significant positive effect on satisfaction and an indirect effect on intent to stay. Recommendations included implementation of a shared decision-making structure to allow nurses to identify sources of job stress and help design effective mitigation strategies.[21]

The component stress and workload received the next to lowest satisfaction score with a mean of 2.63. Analysis of the individual prompts revealed the prompt, "I am able to meet the demands of my job" with a high mean of 4.51. This finding seemed contrary to the low overall mean for the component and the low means for the other 4 individual item prompts. A possible explanation for this finding is that, although the nurses report feeling overwhelmed with their workload, they are able to get their job done and meet the demands, although it may take extra time. They may have thought that saying they cannot meet the demands of their job would indicate a poor level of care or job performance. The 2 lowest mean scores in the category were related to the individual item prompts "At times, I am overwhelmed by all of the work I have to do" (1.57) and "I could deliver better patient care if I had more time," (1.69). Comments relating to stress and workload consistently and overwhelmingly identified the issues of uncompensated time and documentation or computer system. The issue of uncompensated time is documented in the literature. Narayan[5] identified nurses' concern of productivity requirements necessitating 10-hour work days while only being paid for 8. Nurses at the agency identified documentation requirements, nonvisit activities, and patient load or acuity as the contributors to uncompensated time. Dissatisfaction related to stress and workload and excessive paperwork or documentation is well documented in the literature.[12,13,16,21]

The component of job satisfaction with the lowest mean score (2.60) was salary and benefits. The highest mean score among the individual item prompts for this component related to, "The benefit package at this agency is satisfactory to me" (3.47). The lowest mean satisfaction score (1.67) related to, "An upgrade of the pay scales at this agency is needed." Comments related to salary were consistently qualified with the number of hours worked. This finding indicates that the hourly wage or salary is not the sole issue. The issue with pay is that the nurses think they are not paid for the number of hours required to complete the day's work. Dissatisfaction with salary is also well documented in the literature.[12,13,16,21] Comments relating to salary and benefits were overwhelmingly identified as barriers. Most of these barriers (69%) related to the theme uncompensated time, whereas the remaining barriers related to the theme benefits.

Implications and Recommendations

The survey findings have implications for the agency and the home health industry as well as current home health nurses and nurses looking toward a career in home health. The facilitators and barriers to satisfaction for home health nurses revealed in this survey process have been substantiated in the literature for years. To meet the future demands for home health care, job satisfaction of home health nurses must be addressed and improved. Current home health nurses can lead from the point of care by supporting the need for agencies to measure home health nursing job satisfaction and act to remove the barriers and protect and enhance the facilitators to improve job satisfaction and retention. Nurses considering home health as a future career can seek agencies that have high retention and job satisfaction rates.

More current research relating to job satisfaction of home health nurses is needed. Future improvement work in this area should include documentation of the impact of job satisfaction of home health nurses on quality of care and patient satisfaction. Medicare-certified home health agencies are evaluated by CMS and will soon be reimbursed related to quality. With value-based purchasing for home health agencies on the horizon, job satisfaction of the nurses may have an impact on reimbursement. Investigating the impact of strategies implemented to increase job satisfaction of home health nurses is needed.

Home health nurses can advocate for organizational change to improve the level of job satisfaction. Recommendations to improve the level of satisfaction with the components relationship with organization, stress and workload, and salary and benefits and remove the barriers uncompensated time and documentation or the computer system are:

1. Adopt lean management strategies to identify and remove waste and inefficiencies from RN processes.
2. Evaluate current productivity expectations to determine whether the expectations are reasonable, whether all patient care related activities are accounted for, and whether the agency is aligned with the market.
3. Implement incentives to increase availability of as-needed nurses in order to decrease overload of full-time nurses.
4. Identify and implement strategies to streamline and simplify documentation.
5. Evaluate RN salaries and visit rate to determine whether the agency is aligned with the market and whether nurses are being paid for hours worked.
6. Develop and implement a shared governance model.
7. Solicit and consider suggestions made by home health staff nurses.

Recommendations to protect and enhance the levels of higher satisfaction with the components relationship with patients, relationship with peers, and autonomy and control and maximize the facilitators flexibility, one-on-one patient care or patient relationships, management or supervisor, and peers include:

1. Strengthen the case management model to maximize nurse continuity.
2. Implement processes to maximize nurse autonomy, independence, and flexibility.
3. Provide opportunities for peer interactions.
4. Recognize the positive impact of leadership, management, and supervisors.
5. Evaluate and consider the suggestions made by the respondents to the survey.

Recommendations to improve overall job satisfaction include:

1. Measure RN turnover and job satisfaction specific to the RNs on a regular basis to track and evaluate trends, assess effectiveness of strategies, and identify emerging issues.
2. Use the HHNJS scale.[23]
3. Adopt a framework to guide improvement of overall job satisfaction.
4. Investigate the feasibility of implementing a home health nurse residency program.[24]
5. Implement interview questions targeted at choosing nurses who are most likely to succeed and be productive, long-term home health nurses.[25]
6. Highlight and develop the aspects of home health that appeal to the millennial generation. By 2025, 39.4% of nurses will be less than 35 years of age.[26]

The recommendations made for this agency to consider are useful to share with other home health leaders. Professional organizations for the home health industry should consider the development of tool kits based on these recommendations to assist agencies with improving the job satisfaction of home health nurses. Overall job satisfaction of home health nurses is composed of the 8 components identified in the HHNJS, and the HHNJS survey tool is a constructive way to periodically assess RN satisfaction. It is recommended that home health leaders measure satisfaction and address the areas with low scores while enhancing the areas with high scores. Identified facilitators should be protected while steps are taken to remove the identified barriers.

SUMMARY

Home health nurses are highly satisfied with their relationships with patients and peers and the autonomy and control in their jobs. The literature and data presented from the quality improvement process at 1 home health agency identify that home health nurses are least satisfied with their relationships with the organization, the stress and workload, and their salaries and benefits. The strongest, most consistent barrier themes identified were uncompensated time and documentation or computer system. These barrier themes also often impede or minimize facilitators. Based on the results of this satisfaction survey, leaders at this agency made changes in the documentation system and are using results to inform recommendations to be included in an agency retention plan.

Although this examination of 1 agency is limited in scope, the quality improvement and survey process was useful for the leaders in that organization and can serve to inform other home health leaders. This process can easily be replicated by other agencies in order to measure job satisfaction and identify specific areas that are affecting turnover. Further evaluation of job satisfaction of home health nurses and the effectiveness of strategies to enhance facilitators and mitigate barriers is needed. The true financial impact of high RN turnover and low job satisfaction must be analyzed and weighed against the costs of strategies to decrease uncompensated time. Turnover and low job satisfaction can potentially affect patient satisfaction, quality of care, and the ability of agencies to meet the growing need for home health nurses.

ACKNOWLEDGMENTS

The author would like to acknowledge Dr Kimberly Van Haitsma, Dr Kelly A. Wolgast, and Dr Kristen A. Altdoerffer for assistance, guidance, and support with the original DNP quality improvement project that preceded this article. In addition, the author would like to thank Dr Carol Ellenbecker for granting permission to use her HHNJS survey for this project and for providing guidance along the way.

DISCLOSURE

The author has no relevant financial relationship with any commercial companies that have a direct financial interest in subject matter or materials discussed in this article or with any companies making any competing products.

REFERENCES

1. U.S. Department of Labor Bureau of Labor Statistics. Career outlook: projections of industry employment, 2014-2024. 2015. Available at: http://www.bls.gov/careeroutlook/2015/article/projections-industry.htm. Accessed May 29, 2019.
2. U.S. Department of Labor Bureau of Labor statistics. Employment by industry, occupation, and percent distribution, 2016 and projected 2026 home healthcare services. 2017. Available at: https://www.bls.gov/emp/tables/industry-occupation-matrix-industry.htm. Accessed May 29, 2019.
3. Cushman M, Ellenbecker CH. Home care nurse shortage 2007. Caring 2008; 27(1):42–7.
4. Tullai-McGuinness S. Home healthcare practice environment: predictors of RN satisfaction. Res Nurs Health 2008;31(3):252–60.
5. Narayan MC. Survey highlights the concerns of home health nurses. Home Healthc Nurse 1999;17(1):57.
6. Humphrey CJ. Home healthcare nurses forum held at NAHC meeting. Home Healthc Nurse 2003;21(12):791–2.
7. Oregon Center for Nursing. Nurses wanted: the changing demand for registered nurses in Oregon. Portland (OR): Oregon Center for Nursing; 2011.
8. Nursing Solutions, Inc. 2017 National health care retention & RN staffing report. East Petersburg (PA): Nursing Solutions Inc; 2017.

9. Hospital and Healthcare Compensation Service. Home care salary and benefits report 2017-2018. Oakland (NJ): Hospital and Healthcare Compensation Service; 2017.

10. Simmons BL, Nelson DL, Neal LJ. A comparison of the positive and negative work attitudes of home health care and hospital nurses. Health Care Manage Rev 2001;26(3):63–74.

11. Sochalski J. Building a home healthcare workforce to meet the quality imperative. J Healthc Qual 2004;26(3):19–23.

12. Anthony A, Milone-Nuzzo P. Factors attracting and keeping nurses in home care. Home Healthc Nurse 2005;23(6):372–7.

13. Ellenbecker CH, Byleckie JJ. Agencies make a difference in home healthcare nurses' job satisfaction. Home Healthc Nurse 2005;23(12):777–86.

14. Smith-Stoner M. Home care nurses' perceptions of agency and supervisory characteristics: working in the rain. Home Healthc Nurse 2004;22(8):536–46.

15. Ellenbecker CH, Samia L, Cushman MJ, et al. Employer retention strategies and their effect on nurses' job satisfaction and intent to stay. Home Health Care Serv Q 2007;26(1):43–58.

16. Ellenbecker CH, Boylan LN, Samia L. What home healthcare nurses are saying about their jobs. Home Healthc Nurse 2006;24(5):315–24.

17. Smith-Stoner M. There's still no place like home: results of the Home Healthcare Nurse 2002 survey of nurses working in home care and hospice for 20+ years. Home Healthc Nurse 2002;20(10):657–62.

18. Tourangeau A, Patterson E, Rowe A, et al. Factors influencing home care nurse intention to remain employed. J Nurs Manag 2014;22(8):1015–26.

19. Link SH. Statewide home health and hospice nursing survey results. Tualatin (OR): Oregon Nurse; 2009. p. 8.

20. Neal-Boylan L. An analysis of the differences between hospital and home healthcare nurse job satisfaction. Home Healthc Nurse 2006;24(8):505–12.

21. Ellenbecker CH, Cushman M. Home healthcare nurse retention and patient outcome model: discussion and model development. J Adv Nurs 2012;68(8): 1881–93.

22. Smith-Stoner M, Markley J. Home healthcare nurse recruitment and retention: tips for retaining nurses: one state's experience. Home Healthc Nurse 2007;25(3): 198–205.

23. Ellenbecker CH, Byleckie JJ, Samia LW. Further psychometric testing of the home healthcare nurse job satisfaction scale. Res Nurs Health 2008;31(2):152–64.

24. Pittman P, Horton K, Terry M, et al. Residency programs for home health and hospice nurses: prevalence, barriers, and potential policy responses. Home Health Care Manag Pract 2014;26(2):86–91.

25. Mitchell LJ, Oermann M. Hiring and retaining home care nurses. Home Healthc Now 2017;35(1):43–7.

26. Auerbach DI, Chattopadhyay A, Zangaro G, et al. Improving nursing workforce forecasts: comparative analysis of the cohort supply model and the health workforce simulation model. Nurs Econ 2017;35(6):283–326.

Moving?

Make sure your subscription moves with you!

To notify us of your new address, find your **Clinics Account Number** (located on your mailing label above your name), and contact customer service at:

Email: journalscustomerservice-usa@elsevier.com

800-654-2452 (subscribers in the U.S. & Canada)
314-447-8871 (subscribers outside of the U.S. & Canada)

Fax number: 314-447-8029

Elsevier Health Sciences Division
Subscription Customer Service
3251 Riverport Lane
Maryland Heights, MO 63043

*To ensure uninterrupted delivery of your subscription, please notify us at least 4 weeks in advance of move.